OCCUPATIONAL THERAPY EVALUATION FOR ADULTS:
A Pocket Guide

OCCUPATIONAL THERAPY EVALUATION FOR ADULTS
A Pocket Guide

MAUREEN E. NEISTADT
SCD, OTR/L, FAOTA

Acquisition Editor: Margaret Biblis
Managing Editor: Ulita Lushnycky
Marketing Manager: Debby Hartman
Production Editor: Lisa Franko

351 West Camden Street
Baltimore, Maryland 21201-2436 USA

227 East Washington Square
Philadelphia, Pennsylvania 19106 USA

Printed in the United States of America.

Library of Congress Cataloging-in-Publication Data

Neistadt, Maureen E.
    Occupational therapy evaluation for adults : a pocket guide / Maureen E. Neistadt.
      p. cm.
    Includes index.
    ISBN-13 978-0-7817-2495-1
    ISBN-10 0-7817-2495-3
    1. Occupational therapy—Handbooks, manuals, etc. I. Title.

RM735.3 .N45 2000
615.8'515—dc21   00-042130

7 8 9 10

ACKNOWLEDGMENTS

As with any project, this book would not have been possible without the generosity of others. I am grateful to everyone who helped me with this book. Many colleagues and publishers agreed to allow reprints of all or parts of the assessments in this book. Several colleagues—Alexis Henry, ScD, OTR/L, FAOTA, Margo Holm, PhD, OTR/L, FAOTA, ABDA, Kirsten Kohlmeyer, MS, OTR/L, and Joan Rogers, PhD, OTR/L, FAOTA—gave permission to reprint large sections of their work from the 9th edition of *Willard & Spackman's Occupational Therapy* in the appendices of this book.

Pamela Roberts, MSHA, OTR, and the entire occupational therapy department at Cedars-Sinai Medical Center in Los Angeles gave of their time to recruit and photograph clients for some of the pictures in this book. The clients who volunteered gave generously of their time as well. Several senior students in the occupational therapy department at the University of New Hampshire (UNH)—Julie Anderson, Jessica Collins, and Katie Tinkham—also volunteered their time to pose for some of the book's photos. Ron Bergeron and the photo department at UNH made these photo shoots fun and turned around beautiful proofs in record time.

Several colleagues reviewed early drafts of this book and offered valuable suggestions. I would especially like to thank Mary Evenson, MPH, OTR, Pamela Roberts, MSHA, OTR, Cynthia Tufts, OTR/L, and Dorothy Lavoie, OTR/L, for their insights about content novice therapists might find helpful. Elizabeth Crepeau, PhD, OTR/L, FAOTA, has offered constant support and encouragement—both personally and professionally throughout this project.

Margaret Biblis, Executive Editor, Health Professions, at Lippincott Williams and Wilkins (LWW), understood my vision for this book and helped me take if from concept to reality. The reviewers in that process offered careful feedback that helped shape the book. Ulita Lushnycky, Associate Managing Editor at LWW, has offered her careful attention to details throughout the process of getting this book to press.

I would also like to thank my husband Jerry, and my parents, Phyllis and Francis Purcell, for their unfailing interest in this project, and for their love—which has made all things possible.

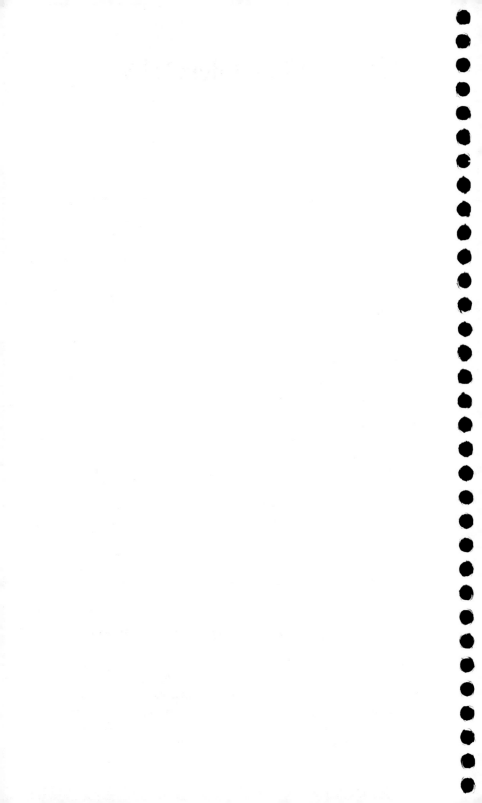

CONTENTS

CHAPTER 1
OCCUPATIONAL THERAPY EVALUATION

CHAPTER 2
A GUIDE TO EVALUATION

Steps:

CHAPTER 3
SUGGESTED EVALUATION SEQUENCES
FOR DIFFERENT TIME LIMITS

APPENDICES

TABLES

CHAPTER 3

BOXES

FIGURES

CHAPTER 2

APPENDIX A

APPENDIX B

APPENDIX C

APPENDIX D

APPENDIX E

APPENDIX G

APPENDIX H

1

OCCUPATIONAL THERAPY EVALUATION

Occupational therapy evaluation is both a set of procedures and a thought process. Evaluation procedures for adults include interviews, activity of daily living (ADL) assessments, and hands-on tests for skills like muscle strength and passive range of motion. The evaluation thought process is a mental set of constantly observing and interpreting clients' behaviors to get an ever-clearer picture of clients' problems and helpful interventions. Evaluation procedures take place within prescribed time periods. As an occupational therapist, you will engage in the evaluation thought process during evaluation procedures AND during all other interactions with clients; that is, occupational therapy practitioners are always evaluating clients' problems and progress during intervention sessions. The evaluation thought process is ongoing from the first through the last meeting with clients.

RELATION BETWEEN EVALUATION, THEORY, AND FRAME OF REFERENCE

Whether you are an occupational therapy student or practitioner, you come to this book with your own ideas about what occupational therapy is and how it should be done. These ideas are linked together to form conceptual structures that (a) help you make sense of your profession and (b) guide your actions as a practitioner. When your ideas are loosely organized, you have a frame of reference. When your ideas are tightly organized, with articulated assumptions and predictions of behavior based on your concepts, you have a theory (Rogers, 1985).

Your frame of reference may be unique to you; it may be a collection of ideas drawn from several theories and frames of reference—ideas that fit together logically in your mind. Frames of reference that draw from several occupational therapy theories and frames of reference are termed "eclectic." Eclectic frames of reference are often tacit, that is, not explicitly articulated (Rogers, 1985). Even when they are tacit, these frames of reference still influence the way you practice, interpret clients' behaviors, interact with clients and families, and relate to other professionals. Therefore, it is important that you spend some time thinking about your ideas relative to occupational therapy practice. If you articulate your personal frame of reference, then you will be more self-aware about the way you make decisions about client care. Being aware of your mindset about occupational therapy evaluation and intervention will make it easier for you to see when your ideas get in your way—by limiting your perceptions and your ideas about intervention options for clients.

You may also find that you modify your frame of reference or use different frames of reference and theories in different situations. Most practitioners engage in this kind of mental flexibility, looking for the best fit between a particular client situation and a conceptual framework to best illuminate that situation.

In writing this book, I have used what I call a general, generic frame of reference for occupational therapy. This general frame of reference focuses on the importance of occupation, client-centered evaluation and intervention, and collaborative therapeutic relationships. Throughout this book, I have looked for ways to make occupation and client-centered evaluation work within healthcare systems that focus on efficient and expedient service delivery.

EVALUATION AND CLINICAL REASONING

Your personal frame of reference helps to organize your approach to evaluation. Within that conceptual framework, you will use multiple types of clinical reasoning during the evaluation thought process. "Clinical reasoning" is neither a frame of reference nor a new approach to client care. It is simply a description of how occupational therapy (OT) practitioners think no matter what their frame of reference. The thought processes described by clinical reasoning terms are not new; OT practitioners have always thought this way. The language of clinical reasoning is relatively new to the field; it was first articulated in Joan Rogers' work in the early 1980s and has continued to evolve since then (e.g., Mattingly & Fleming, 1994; Rogers, 1983; Rogers & Masagatani, 1982; Schell & Cervero, 1993). Having descriptive labels for your different types of thinking can help you to become more aware of how you are thinking and to articulate thought processes that have become automatic. In articulating these thought processes, you come to appreciate the complexity of your thinking and gain insight into ways to improve your thinking. Table 1-1 defines these different types of clinical reasoning and shows how they are used during evaluation and intervention.

Your occupational therapy evaluation and intervention will be most effective and efficient when you use narrative reasoning to make the client's life story and priorities the focus and general background of all other types of reasoning, that is, when you think first about working with a person, not a set of problems. Consequently, the evaluation sequence suggested in Chapter 2 is client-centered and uses narrative reasoning throughout to illuminate clients' valued activities and perceptions of their difficulties.

Chapter 2 also suggests you focus your procedural reasoning on a top-down approach to evaluation. The top down approach starts with observation of clients' valued activities or occupational performance areas. You use activity analysis during this observation to generate hypotheses about what impairments or occupational component skill deficits might be contributing to difficulties in functional activity performance. These hypotheses can then be tested with formal evaluation of the targeted component skill areas.

This top-down approach is client-centered and helps you do the following: (a) immediately identify functional performance problems of concern to clients, and (b) focus quickly on those component skills that appear problematic. Occupational therapy's most important contribution to client care is a delineation of the client's functional problems and priorities. Focusing on the most relevant component skills makes evaluation more efficient. This efficiency is vital in today's health care market.

DEMANDS OF THE HEALTHCARE MARKETPLACE

In the past, third-party payers in the United States reimbursed occupational therapists for any and all evaluations the therapists felt were necessary, no matter how much time those procedures took. The duration of intervention was also left largely to the discretion of therapists. Now third-party payers are limiting their reimbursement for evaluation and intervention time, refusing payment for evaluation or intervention time that exceeds given limits. The amount of time allowed for evaluation or intervention will vary from payer to payer. In some cases, a therapist's first visit with a client will not be reimbursed at all unless that first visit includes intervention time along with evaluation time.

TABLE 1-1 | TYPES OF CLINICAL REASONING USED DURING EVALUATION

Type of Clinical Reasoning	Definition	Practitioner Actions	Contribution to the Evaluation and Intervention Process
Narrative Reasoning	Yields the client's occupational story, i.e., his or her life history as told through preferred activities, habits, and roles. Also encompasses the client's and therapist's story together, i.e., how the therapist and client will incorporate the client's activity preferences into intervention to build a meaningful future for the client.	Interview about clients' routine activities, activity priorities, social, vocational, and educational history	Focus on client goals leads to efficient evaluation and intervention Focus on client goals increases client motivation and participation in therapy
Interactive Reasoning	Yields an understanding of what the disease or disability means to the client, i.e., the client's illness experience. Also encompasses the interpersonal interactions between therapists and clients.	Therapeutic use of self, working collaboratively with clients	Taps client motivation and increases learning; increases client satisfaction; decreases client anxiety
Procedural Reasoning	The process of defining clients' diagnostically related problems with (a) their routine life activities, (b) the skills that contribute to those activities, and (c) the environments in which those activities occur, and selecting appropriate interventions.	Evaluation procedures and assessments, activity analysis, use of activity as a therapeutic modality	Identification of clients' OT problems and of interventions appropriate to those problems

Pragmatic Reasoning	Used to consider all of the practical issues that affect occupational therapy services: the intervention environment; the therapist's values, knowledge, abilities, and experiences; clients' social and financial resources; clients' potential discharge environments.	Ongoing monitoring of insurance coverage, own knowledge base, effects of the environment on clients, and clients' resources	Identification of best intervention in any particular setting; discharge projections
Ethical Reasoning	Used to choose a morally defensible course of action with clients, in the face of competing interests.	Ongoing attention to client's goals and their relation to goals of caregivers and providers	Identification of ethical intervention for any given client
Conditional Reasoning	Used to revise intervention moment to moment to meet clients' needs. This revision is done with an eye to clients' current and possible future contexts.	Flexibility regarding therapy agenda in any particular session	Increases client participation; highlights importance of activity analysis to discover therapeutic potential of all activities

Note: Complied from Mattingly & Fleming, 1994; Schell, 1998; Schell & Cervero, 1993.

In some facilities, support staff or case managers will help you keep track of therapy limits for your clients. In other cases, you will need to keep track of this information yourself. In some settings, you will need to obtain prior approval from a third-party payer before you can begin working with a client. Check with your supervisor when you begin a new job to learn what your responsibilities are in that setting regarding checking the client's insurance coverage for therapy.

As a result of these reimbursement changes, occupational therapy practitioners in the United States now have less time to work with clients than ever before. This means you need to use your theories and frames of reference to prioritize both evaluation and intervention procedures, to ensure clients' maximal benefit from the limited therapy time permitted by their third-party payers. The shorter allowable times for evaluation may also mean you will need to rely on observation and interpretation of clients' behavior more heavily than on formal evaluation procedures to determine clients' problems and possible solutions.

Shorter evaluation times also mean you will need to be using more screening techniques. "Screening involves a cursory evaluation to determine if a more intensive evaluation is needed" (Rogers & Holm, 1998, p. 186). Your theories and frames of reference can help you decide when to use screenings to quickly check for the presence or absence of problems, as well as when to perform more detailed formal procedures for problems that arise during screenings.

INFORMATION NEEDED FROM SCREENING AND EVALUATION

Box 1-1 delineates the information your initial screening and evaluation should yield. Table 1-2 lists some client strengths and notes how those might affect the intervention process.

Ongoing evaluation during intervention can supplement the information you gather initially. You will use conditional reasoning to work new information into the intervention plan and modify intervention as needed while you and the client work together toward mutual goals.

SUGGESTIONS FOR USE OF THE REST OF THE BOOK

Chapter 2 provides brief guidelines for an evaluation process, organized by the steps you will follow during an evaluation. Again, the frame

BOX 1-1	INFORMATION NEEDED FROM INITIAL OCCUPATIONAL THERAPY SCREENING AND EVALUATION

1) A list of specific client activity priorities, i.e., specific activities the client needs and wants to be able to do
2) A narrative summary of client strengths, i.e., personal assets the client brings to the intervention process (see first paragraph of Box 2-6 for an example)
3) A list of client problems in:
   - Basic Activities of Daily Living (BADL) or self-care
   - Instrumental Activities of Daily Living (IADL) or community living skills
   - Component skills contributing to ADL difficulties
   - Living environments
4) A discharge projection (projected BADL and IADL skill levels and living situation), determined in collaboration with the client and his or her caregivers
5) An intervention plan to achieve the discharge projections, which is also determined in collaboration with the client and his or her caregivers

TABLE 1-2	SOME CLIENT STRENGTHS AND THEIR RELEVANCE FOR INTERVENTION PROCESS

Client Strength Phrased Appropriately for Documentation	Potential Contribution to Intervention Process
Knowledgeable about own disease or disability	Client will not need extensive education about his or her disease or disability, will be able to contribute actively to brainstorming with practitioner about adaptive strategies for BADL and IADL
Able to learn quickly	Client will be able to grasp and apply the concepts behind adaptive techniques quickly
Energetic, involved in process of own care	Client will follow through with intervention program on own
Supportive family and/or friends	Family and friends may be able to help client post discharge
Owns home or has landlord willing to make environmental adaptations	Reasonable cost adaptations to current living quarters can be made as needed

of reference underlying this organization views occupational therapy as a client-centered process most appropriately focused on occupation. Chapter 2 is meant to help you organize and access all of the information you learned in school about occupational therapy evaluation. Appendices A through G, cited throughout Chapter 2, provide additional detail about specific evaluation procedures, for quick reference; these appendices also include ordering information for assessments and evaluation materials.

Chapter 3 suggests evaluation sequences for different time limits. These different sequences should help you plan evaluations that are comprehensive yet realistic for your time constraints.

Appendices H and I provide details about the American Occupational Therapy Association's Occupational Therapy Uniform and the World Health Organizations International Classification of Impairments, Disability, and Handicaps-2 terminology. These appendices are included to help you be precise in your use of terminology for whichever terminology your setting prefers.

2
A GUIDE TO EVALUATION

STEPS

Evaluation is the process of gathering and interpreting information about clients to determine their needs for occupational therapy services. This process is summarized in the Evaluation checklist in Box 2-1. The following text provides detail about each of the steps in that checklist.

STEP 1 Review the client's medical record and/or other pre-evaluation information.

The level of pre-evaluation information available to you will vary from setting to setting. In some situations, you will have access to the client's medical and social history. In other situations, the only pre-evaluation information you have is a general occupational therapy order such as "OT eval and treat" or "ADL eval and treat," along with the name, age, and gender of the client. When complete client records are not available, you will have to rely on the client and his or her caregivers to explain the problems behind this OT referral. If the client and caregivers are confused about the nature of the problems, you will need to call the referral source for clarification and additional information. At the very least, you should ask the referral source for a diagnosis or specific description of the problems that triggered the referral.

The client's diagnosis can give you a preliminary idea of (a) what precautions need to be observed when working with the client and (b) what types of diagnosis-related OT problems the client might be experiencing. For example, a client with cardiovascular disease might (a) be at risk for cardiac arrest with overexertion and (b) have severe en-

BOX 2-1	EVALUATION CHECKLIST

Review the client's medical record and/or other pre-evaluation information.

____ Collect your evaluation materials.

____ Check with nursing to see if the client can be seen.

____ Stop before entering the client's space, take a deep breath, clear your mind, and focus on taking in everything you will see and hear during your evaluation.

____ Knock before entering client's room, home, or space.

____ Read any signs posted in client's environment about medical precautions or care procedures.

____ Introduce yourself, ask the client how he or she would like to be addressed, and make sure the client is physically comfortable.

____ Interview the client and/or his or her caregivers.

____ Observe functional performance and record observations.

____ Evaluate component skills contributing to functional performance problems and record evaluation results.

____ Note type and amount of cuing client needs for activity performance.

____ Synthesize and summarize the data; make discharge projections— project and record rehabilitation objectives and interventions planned to reach discharge projections.

durance problems that negatively affect the performance of all routine activities. You use procedural reasoning to make the links between diagnosis and potential precautions and OT problems. Box 2-2 lists major precautions related to client and practitioner safety for several diagnoses and client problems.

The pre-evaluation information might also provide some initial information about the client's social history and potential discharge situation. You use narrative reasoning to think about this information, to begin understanding (a) how this client's life story has been changed by the problems that have brought him or her to occupational therapy and (b) how the client's life story might play out in the future given his or her current problems.

STEP 2   Collect your evaluation materials.

Before you see a client, you need to have your evaluation materials organized. A notebook might be useful for frequently used forms. A canvas bag could be used to carry additional evaluation materials for

BOX 2-2	PRECAUTIONS RELATED TO CLIENT AND PRACTITIONER SAFETY

■ Activity restrictions owing to cardiovascular disease (e.g., myocardial infarction [MI] or deep vein thrombosis [DVT])

  * Know safe vital sign limits for clients with cardiovascular disease—these will be individual and should be checked with the client's physician. The following are general guidelines only and will not apply to all clients.

  Pulse or heart rate (HR)—typically, a safe HR limit is an increase of no more than 20–30 beats per minute (bpm) above resting rate. If HR is less than 50 in response to activity, activity should be stopped, and a physician or nursing staff contacted.

  Blood Pressure (BP)—typically, a safe BP limit is an increase or decrease of no more than 15–20 mm Hg from resting.

  Respiratory Rate (RR)—monitor client for shortness of breath.

  * Monitor client for signs of cardiovascular distress—sweating, pallor, nausea, pain in left arm or jaw, chest pain, or dizziness.

  * Moving clients with DVT could dislodge their thrombosis causing an MI, respiratory arrest, or a stroke.

■ Activity restrictions owing to pulmonary disease (e.g., chronic obstructive pulmonary disease [COPD])

  * Use oximeter if available—know safe oxygen saturation levels for particular client.

  * Monitor for signs of respiratory distress—shortness of breath, sweating, pallor, or dizziness.

■ Careful moving of client so as not to dislodge medical equipment and indwelling tubes (e.g., respirators and urinary catheters).

■ Possible seizure activity with neurologic diagnoses (e.g., stroke or traumatic brain injury)

■ Universal infection precautions with all clients

■ Falls precautions for clients with balance problems

  * Always have client wear shoes for walking or being transferred.

  * Keep working area well-lit (to compensate for decreased visual acuity).

  * Reduce glare from sunlight, bright lights, and shiny surfaces as much as possible (task lighting; no wax on furniture; no glare wax on floors; use sheer curtains, blinds, and drapes; do not have client face direct sunlight).

  * Be aware of the decreased ability to accommodate to light changes in older adults (use night lights; have light switches and lamps at entrances to rooms; have client pause before moving from one lighting condition to another, e.g., from bright hallway to darker room, to allow eyes time to adjust to new lighting condition).

CHAPTER 2

home-based or bedside evaluations. Table 2-1 defines the types of evaluation procedures that are available; however, the exact combination of these that you use will depend on your practice setting and the amount of time you have for your evaluation.

The client's diagnosis or referring problem will give you a general idea of what evaluation procedures and assessments might be appropriate. Tables 2-2 through 2-9 provide some examples; you will need

TABLE 2-1	TYPES OF EVALUATION PROCEDURES		
Type	**Definition**	**Examples**	**What You Will Need**
Assessments	Standardized instruments used in the evaluation process. These instruments have generally been studied re: their reliability and validity.	Functional Independence Measure (FIM) Lowenstein Occupational Therapy Cognitive (LOTCA) Evaluation	Forms and any testing materials that come with the assessment
Formal Procedures	Procedures have structured guidelines that different therapists may modify. There is usually no reliability or validity data available on these types of procedures.	Manual Muscle Testing (MMT) Goniometry	Forms, necessary tools (e.g., goniometer), any instructions you might want to refer to during the testing. Sharing your instructions or manuals with clients helps them to understand the evaluation procedures and is a good mechanism for client education.
Observation	Practitioner watches client actions and listens to client verbalizations.	Quality of client's movements during Basic & Instrumental Activities of Daily Living (BADL & LADL) Client's verbal and nonverbal responses to interview questions	Forms for guiding and recording observations

to pick and choose from these tables, considering your practice setting, the evaluation materials available, and the time you have to evaluate your client. You should mentally review those procedures and assessments you plan to use, understanding that you may have to change your evaluation plan once you actually meet the client. Pre-evaluation information never gives you a complete picture of the client's medical or mental status. Therefore, the exact combination of evaluation procedures you use may vary from client to client—even for those clients with similar diagnoses.

STEP 3   Check with nursing to see if the client can be seen.

In practice settings in which you work with nurses, check with the nursing staff before you go to see a client to be certain the client is not too ill to be seen for an occupational therapy evaluation.

STEP 4   Stop before entering the client's space, take a deep breath, clear your mind, and focus on taking in everything you will see and hear during your evaluation.

During an evaluation, you need to be alert to the client's verbal and nonverbal communication, the client's movements, the evaluation environment, and the ways the environment affects the client's behavior. You cannot take in all of this information if you are distracted by thoughts about how well you will do this evaluation or about other things you have to do during the workday. Stopping to take a few deep breaths before you enter the client's space will help you to clear your mind of distracting thoughts and focus your attention on the client and his or her surroundings. With your attention focused, you will be able to truly be there with the client during your evaluation.

STEP 5   Knock before entering the client's room, home, or space.

You would not think to barge into a person's home without knocking. But you might not think to knock before you enter a client's room in a hospital setting. Barging into a client's room or space without knocking is just as rude and inconsiderate as barging into someone's home without knocking. In a hospital or nursing home setting, the client's bed, bureau, and closet are his or her living space and you should never enter that space without permission. Even if a client is comatose, you (text continues on page 30)

CHAPTER 2

TABLE 2-2	SUGGESTED EVALUATION PROCEDURES AND ASSESSMENTS FOR CLIENTS WITH NEUROLOGICAL DIAGNOSES AFFECTING THE BRAIN OR SPINAL CORD

Evaluation Area	Assessments	Procedures	Observations
Client priorities and life story	■ Canadian Occupational Performance Measure (COPM)	■ Informal interview ■ Interest Checklists	
Basic Activities of Daily Living (BADL) or self-care	■ Functional Independence Measure (FIM) ■ Arnadottir OT-ADL Neurobehavioral Evaluation (A-ONE) ■ Klein-Bell Activities of Daily Living Scale (Klein-Bell) ■ Performance Assessment of Self-Care Skills (PASS)	BADL rated with scale developed by facility or agency	Use activity analysis to hypothesize component skill deficits underlying performance problems
Instrumental Activities of Daily Living (IADL) or community living skills	■ Rabideau Kitchen Evaluation-Revised (RKE-R) ■ Kohlman Evaluation of Living Skills (KELS) ■ Satisfaction with Performance Scaled Questionnaire (SPSQ) ■ Assessment of Living Skills and Resources (ALSAR) ■ Assessment of Motor and Process Skills (AMPS)	Community living skills rated with scale developed by facility or agency	Use activity analysis to hypothesize component skill deficits underlying performance problems
Sensory skills		Visual screening Somatic sensory testing Oral sensation if swallowing is a problem	Observation of sensory behaviors during functional tasks (e.g. sensitivity to hot & cold water during bathing)

Perceptual/Cognitive skills	Lowenstein Occupational Therapy Cognitive Evaluation (LOTCA) Test of orientation for Rehabilitation Patients (TORP)	Mini-Mental State (MMS)	Observation of perceptual/cognitive skills during functional activities
Motor skills	■ Functional Reach Test (Balance) ■ Tinetti's balance & gait evaluation (Balance) ■ Nine Hole Peg Test of Coordination	Evaluation of muscle tone Manual Muscle Testing (MMT) for muscles with normal tone Passive Range of Motion (PROM) measurement Soft tissue evaluation Oral motor evaluation if swallowing is a problem	Observation of motor control during functional activities Observation of balance during functional activities
Psychosocial skills			Observation of psychosocial skills during evaluation session(s)
Discharge situation		Home visit with form used by facility or agency Family meetings	

Note. ADL = Activities of Daily Living; OT = occupational therapy; See Appendices A–G and pp. 31–79 for details.

TABLE 2-3	SUGGESTED EVALUATION PROCEDURES AND ASSESSMENTS FOR CLIENTS WITH NEUROLOGICAL DIAGNOSES AFFECTING PERIPHERAL NERVES

Evaluation Area	Assessments	Procedures	Observations
Client priorities and life story	▪ Canadian Occupational Performance Measure (COPM)	▪ Informal interview ▪ Interest Checklists	
Basic Activities of Daily Living (BADL) or self-care	▪ Functional Independence Measure (FIM) ▪ Klein-Bell Activities of Daily Living Scale (Klein-Bell) ▪ Performance Assessment of Self-Care Skills (PASS)	BADL rated with scale developed by facility or agency	Use activity analysis to hypothesize component skill deficits underlying performance problems
Instrumental Activities of Daily Living (IADL) or community living skills	▪ Rabideau Kitchen Evaluation-Revised (RKE-R) ▪ Satisfaction with Performance Scaled Questionnaire (SPSQ) ▪ Worker Role Interview	▪ Community living skills rated with scale developed by facility or agency ▪ Work site evaluation	Use activity analysis to hypothesize component skill deficits underlying performance problems
Sensory skills		Somatic sensory testing	Observation of sensory behaviors during functional tasks (e.g., sensitivity to hot & cold water during bathing)

Perceptual/Cognitive Skills	Not applicable unless client has secondary diagnosis of brain injury	Not applicable unless client has secondary diagnosis of brain injury	Observation of perceptual/cognitive skills during functional activities
Motor skills	■ Functional Reach Test (Balance) ■ Tinetti's balance & gait evaluation (Balance) (Balance tests only needed if peripheral nerve problems affect the legs) ■ Nine Hole Peg Test of Coordination ■ Purdue Pegboard Test (Coordination) ■ Crawford Small Parts Test ■ Grooved Pegboard Test ■ Minnesota Rate of Manipulation Test	Evaluation of muscle tone (looking for low tone in denervated muscles) Manual Muscle Testing (MMT) Passive Range of Motion (PROM) measurement Soft tissue evaluation	Observation of coordination during functional activities Observation of coordination during functional activities Observation of balance during functional activities
Psychosocial skills	Not applicable unless client has secondary diagnosis of brain injury or mental health dysfunction	Not applicable unless client has secondary diagnosis of brain injury or mental health dysfunction	Observation of psychosocial skills during evaluation session(s)
Discharge situation		Home visit with form developed by facility or agency Family meetings	

Note. See Appendices A–G and pp. 31–79 for details.

CHAPTER 2

17

TABLE 2-4 | SUGGESTED EVALUATION PROCEDURES AND ASSESSMENTS FOR CLIENTS WITH ORTHOPEDIC AND MUSCULOSKELETAL DIAGNOSES

Evaluation Area	Assessments	Procedures	Observations
Client priorities and life story	▪ Canadian Occupational Performance Measure (COPM)	▪ Informal interview ▪ Interest Checklists	
Basic Activities of Daily Living (BADL) or self-care	▪ Functional Independence Measure (FIM) ▪ Klein-Bell Activities of Daily Living Scale (Klein-Bell) ▪ Performance Assessment of Self-Care Skills (PASS)	BADL rated with scale developed by facility or agency	Use activity analysis to hypothesize component skill deficits underlying performance problems
Instrumental Activities of Daily Living (IADL) or community living skills	▪ Rabideau Kitchen Evaluation-Revised (RKE-R) ▪ Satisfaction with Performance Scaled Questionnaire (SPSQ) ▪ Worker Role Interview	▪ Community living skills rated with scale developed by facility or agency ▪ Work site evaluation	Use activity analysis to hypothesize component skill deficits underlying performance problems
Sensory skills		Somatic sensory screening	Observation of sensory behaviors during functional tasks (e.g. sensitivity to hot & cold water during bathing)
Perceptual/Cognitive skills	Not applicable unless client has secondary diagnosis of brain injury	Not applicable unless client has secondary diagnosis of brain injury	Observation of perceptual/cognitive skills during functional activities

Motor skills	▪ Functional Reach Test (Balance) ▪ Tinetti's balance & gait evaluation (Balance) (Balance tests only needed if diagnosis affects the trunk or legs) ▪ Nine Hole Peg Test of Coordination ▪ Purdue Pegboard Test (Coordination) ▪ Crawford Small Parts Test ▪ Grooved Pegboard Test ▪ Minnesota Rate of Manipulation Test (Coordination tests only needed if diagnosis affects arms and hands.)	Evaluation of muscle tone for those with musculoskeletal diagnoses Manual Muscle Testing (MMT) Passive Range of Motion (PROM) Soft tissue evaluation	Observation of balance during functional activities Observation of coordination during functional activities
Psychosocial skills	Not applicable unless client has secondary diagnosis of brain injury or mental health dysfunction	Not applicable unless client has secondary diagnosis of brain injury or mental health dysfunction	Observation of psychosocial skills during evaluation session(s)
Discharge situation		Home visit with form developed by facility or agency Family meetings	

Note. See Appendices A–G and pp. 31–79 for details.

TABLE 2-5	SUGGESTED EVALUATION PROCEDURES AND ASSESSMENTS FOR CLIENTS WITH CARDIOPULMONARY DIAGNOSES

Evaluation Area	Assessments	Procedures	Observations
Client priorities and life story	▪ Canadian Occupational Performance Measure (COPM)	▪ Informal interview ▪ Interest Checklists	
Basic Activities of Daily Living (BADL) or self-care	▪ Functional Independence Measure (FIM) ▪ Klein-Bell Activities of Daily Living Scale (Klein-Bell) ▪ Performance Assessment of Self-Care Skills (PASS)	BADL rated with scale developed by facility or agency	Use activity analysis to hypothesize component skill deficits underlying performance problems
Instrumental Activities of Daily Living (IADL) or community living skills	▪ Rabideau Kitchen Evaluation-Revised (RKE-R) ▪ Satisfaction with Performance Scaled Questionnaire (SPSQ) ▪ Worker Role Interview	▪ Community living skills rated with scale developed by facility or agency ▪ Work site evaluation	Use activity analysis to hypothesize component skill deficits underlying performance problems
Sensory skills		Somatic sensory screening	Observation of sensory behaviors during functional tasks (e.g. sensitivity to hot & cold water during bathing)

Perceptual/Cognitive skills	Lowenstein Occupational Therapy Cognitive Evaluation (LOTCA)	Mini-Mental State (MMS)	Observation of perceptual/cognitive skills during functional activities
Motor skills	Vital signs monitoring for endurance at beginning, during and end of session: ■ Blood pressure (BP) ■ Heart rate (HR) ■ Respiratory rate (RR) ■ Oximeter for clients with pulmonary diagnoses to monitor levels of blood oxygen saturation	Active Range of Motion (AROM)/Passive Range of Motion (PROM) screen Manual Muscle Testing (MMT) Activity tolerance Borg Perceived Exertion Scale	Observation of balance during functional activities Observation of coordination during functional activities
Psychosocial skills			Observation of psychosocial skills during evaluation session(s)
Discharge situation		Home visit with form developed by facility or agency Family meetings	

Note. See Appendices A–G and pp. 31–79 for details.

TABLE 2-6	SUGGESTED EVALUATION PROCEDURES AND ASSESSMENTS FOR CLIENTS WITH IMMUNOLOGICAL DISORDERS (E.G., CANCER, HIV INFECTION)

Evaluation Area	Assessments	Procedures	Observations
Client priorities and life story	▪ Canadian Occupational Performance Measure (COPM)	▪ Informal interview ▪ Interest Checklists	
Basic Activities of Daily Living (BADL) or self-care	▪ Functional Independence Measure (FIM) ▪ Arnadottir OT-ADL Neurobehavioral Evaluation (A-ONE) (if brain function affected) ▪ Klein-Bell Activities of Daily Living Scale (Klein-Bell) ▪ Performance Assessment of Self-Care Skills (PASS)	BADL rated with scale developed by facility or agency	Use activity analysis to hypothesize component skill deficits underlying performance problems
Instrumental Activities of Daily Living (IADL) or community living skills	▪ Kohlman Evaluation of Living Skills (KELS) ▪ Satisfaction with Performance Scaled Questionnaire (SPSQ) ▪ Assessment of Living Skills and Resources (ALSAR) ▪ Assessment of Motor and Process Skills (AMPS) ▪ Community Integration Questionnaire	Community living skills rated with scale developed by facility or agency	Use activity analysis to hypothesize component skill deficits underlying performance problems
Sensory skills		Visual screening Somatic sensory screening	Observation of sensory behaviors during functional tasks (e.g. sensitivity to hot & cold water during bathing) Observation of pain behaviors during functional tasks (grimacing, tensing, guarding a body part)

Perceptual/Cognitive skills	Lowenstein Occupational Therapy Cognitive Evaluation (LOTCA) Test of orientation for Rehabilitation Patients (TORP) (These only if brain function is affected)	Mini-Mental State (MMS) (if brain function is affected)	Observation of perceptual/cognitive skills during functional activities
Motor skills	■ Functional Reach Test (Balance) ■ Tinetti's balance & gait evaluation (Balance) ■ Nine Hole Peg Test of Coordination	Evaluation of muscle tone Manual Muscle Testing (MMT) for muscles with normal tone Passive Range of Motion (PROM) measurement Soft tissue evaluation	Observation of motor control during functional activities Observation of balance during functional activities
Psychosocial skills			Observation of psychosocial skills during evaluation session(s)
Discharge situation		Home visit with form used by facility or agency Family meetings	

Note. ADL = Activities of Daily Living; OT = occupational therapy, See Appendices A–G and pp. 31–79 for details.

TABLE 2-7	SUGGESTED EVALUATION PROCEDURES AND ASSESSMENTS FOR CLIENTS WITH PSYCHOSOCIAL DIAGNOSES

Evaluation Area	Assessments	Procedures	Observations
Client priorities and life story	▪ Canadian Occupational Performance Measure (COPM)	▪ Informal interview ▪ Interest Checklists	
Basic Activities of Daily Living (BADL) or self-care	▪ Performance Assessment of Self-Care Skills (PASS) ▪ Milwaukee Evaluation of Daily Living Skills (MEDLS)	BADL rated with scale developed by facility or agency	Use activity analysis to hypothesize component skill deficits underlying performance problems
Instrumental Activities of Daily Living (IADL) or community living skills	▪ Milwaukee Evaluation of Daily Living Skills (MEDLS) ▪ Kohlman Evaluation of Living Skills (KELS) ▪ Assessment of Motor and Process Skills (AMPS) ▪ Worker Role Interview (WRI)	Community living skills rated with scale developed by facility or agency	Use activity analysis to hypothesize component skill deficits underlying performance problems
Sensory skills		Visual screening if client complains of visual difficulties Somatic sensory screening only if client complains of sensory problems	Observation of sensory behaviors during functional tasks (e.g. sensitivity to hot & cold water during bathing)

Perceptual/Cognitive skills	Lowenstein Occupational Therapy Cognitive Evaluation (LOTCA)	Mini-Mental State (MMS)	Observation of perceptual/cognitive skills during functional activities Note client reports of perceptual disturbances (hallucinations, illusions, depersonalization)
Motor skills	Not appropriate unless client also has motor problems	Not appropriate unless client also has motor problems	Observation of motor control during functional activities Observation of balance during functional activities
Psychosocial skills	Occupational Case Analysis & Interview Rating Scale (OCAIRS) Assessment of Occupational Functioning (AOF) Occupational Performance History Interview II (OPHI II) Role Activity Performance Scale (RAPS) Allen Cognitive Level Test-90 (ACLS-90)		Observation of psychosocial skills during evaluation session(s)
Discharge situation		Home visit with form used by facility or agency Family meetings	

Note. See Appendices A–G and pp. 31–79 for details.

TABLE 2-8	SUGGESTED EVALUATION PROCEDURES AND ASSESSMENTS FOR CLIENTS WITH BURNS

Evaluation Area	Assessments	Procedures	Observations
Client priorities and life story	▪ Canadian Occupational Performance Measure (COPM)	▪ Informal interview ▪ Interest Checklists	
Basic Activities of Daily Living (BADL) or self-care	▪ Functional Independence Measure (FIM) ▪ Klein-Bell Activities of Daily Living Scale (Klein-Bell) ▪ Performance Assessment of Self-Care Skills (PASS)	BADL rated with scale developed by facility or agency	Use activity analysis to hypothesize component skill deficits underlying performance problems
Instrumental Activities of Daily Living (IADL) or community living skills	▪ Kohlman Evaluation of Living Skills (KELS) ▪ Satisfaction with Performance Scaled Questionnaire (SPSQ) ▪ Assessment of Living Skills and Resources (ALSAR) ▪ Community Integration Questionnaire ▪ Worker Role Interview	Community living skills rated with scale developed by facility or agency	Use activity analysis to hypothesize component skill deficits underlying performance problems
Sensory skills		Visual screening Somatic sensory screening	Observation of sensory behaviors during functional tasks (e.g. sensitivity to hot & cold water during bathing) Observation of pain behaviors during functional tasks (grimacing, tensing, guarding a body part)

Perceptual/Cognitive skills	Lowenstein Occupational Therapy Cognitive Evaluation (LOTCA) (These only if brain function is affected)	Mini-Mental State (MMS) (if brain function is affected)	Observation of perceptual/cognitive skills during functional activities
Motor skills	▪ Nine Hole Peg Test of Coordination ▪ Purdue Pegboard Test (Coordination) ▪ Crawford Small Parts Test ▪ Grooved Pegboard Test ▪ Minnesota Rate of Manipulation Test (If burns affect arms and hands)	Evaluation of muscle tone Manual Muscle Testing (MMT) Passive Range of Motion (PROM) measurement Soft tissue evaluation Skin integrity evaluations	Observation of motor control during functional activities Observation of balance during functional activities
Psychosocial skills			Observation of psychosocial skills during evaluation session(s)
Discharge situation		Home visit with form used by facility or agency Family meetings	

Note. See Appendices A–G and pp. 31–79 for details.

27

TABLE 2-9 SUGGESTED EVALUATION PROCEDURES AND ASSESSMENTS FOR CLIENTS REFERRED FOR "ADL EVAL AND TREAT"

Evaluation Area	Assessments	Procedures	Observations
Client priorities and life story	▪ Canadian Occupational Performance Measure (COPM)	▪ Informal interview ▪ Interest Checklists	
Basic Activities of Daily Living (BADL) or self-care	▪ Functional Independence Measure (FIM) ▪ Klein-Bell Activities of Daily Living Scale (Klein-Bell) ▪ Performance Assessment of Self-Care Skills (PASS)	BADL rated with scale developed by facility or agency	Use activity analysis to hypothesize component skill deficits underlying performance problems
Instrumental Activities of Daily Living (IADL) or community living skills	▪ Rabideau Kitchen Evaluation–Revised (RKE-R) ▪ Kohlman Evaluation of Living Skills (KELS) ▪ Satisfaction with Performance Scaled Questionnaire (SPSQ) ▪ Assessment of Living Skills and Resources (ALSAR) ▪ Assessment of Motor and Process Skills (AMPS)	Community living skills rated with scale developed by facility or agency	Use activity analysis to hypothesize component skill deficits underlying performance problems
Sensory skills		Visual screening Somatic sensory screening	Observation of sensory behaviors during functional tasks (e.g. sensitivity to hot & cold water during bathing)

Perceptual/Cognitive skills	Lowenstein Occupational Therapy Cognitive Evaluation (LOTCA) (If perception and cognition are problems)	Mini-Mental State (MMS) (If perception and cognition are problems)	Observation of perceptual/cognitive skills during functional activities
Motor skills	▪ Functional Reach Test (Balance) (if balance is a problem) ▪ Nine Hole Peg Test of Coordination (if coordination is a problem)	Evaluation of muscle tone Manual Muscle Testing (MMT) for muscles with normal tone Passive Range of Motion (PROM) measurement Soft tissue evaluation	Observation of motor control during functional activities Observation of balance during functional activities
Psychosocial skills			Observation of psychosocial skills during evaluation session(s)
Discharge situation		Home visit with form used by facility or agency Family meetings	

Note. ADL = Activities of Daily Living; Assessments for specific component skills would only be appropriate if screening for these areas indicated problems. See Appendices A–G and pp. 31–79 for details of assessments and procedures.

should knock on the door to the room, on the end of the bed, or on a closet door, to acknowledge that you are entering that client's space. You need to get into the habit of showing all clients this respect and consideration.

STEP 6   Read any signs posted in the client's environment about medical precautions or care procedures.

In hospital settings, signs may have been posted about medical equipment, infection precautions, clients' swallowing status, or recommended procedures for transfers and bed mobility. In home situations, signs may have been posted to note clients' usual ADL routines or medication schedules. You are responsible for reading and understanding all signs in a client's environment.

STEP 7   Introduce yourself, ask the client how he or she would like to be addressed, and make sure the client is physically comfortable.

To begin your interactions with the client, you need to introduce yourself and explain the purpose of your visit. If the client is alert, you could start with something such as the introduction in Box 2-3.

You will also need to know how the client would like to be addressed:

"Would you like me to call you [**Mr. or Ms.**] [**client's last name**]?" Do not call the client by his or her first name unless given permission to do so.

BOX 2-3	INTRODUCTION FOR ALERT CLIENT

Hello, I am [**your first and last name**] from occupational therapy. You can call me [**your preference**]. I am here to see if you need any help right now with your day-to-day activities due to your [**client's diagnosis**]. As an occupational therapist, my job is to help you do the daily activities you consider important, despite the problems you are having from your [**client's diagnosis**].

I will begin by asking you a few questions about yourself. Then I will be asking you to move around in bed and get out of bed and to try doing some self-care tasks. I may also be testing the strength, sensation, and joint flexibility in your arms. Does this sound okay to you?

Ask the client if he or she is physically comfortable. If the answer is no, ask if it would be okay for you to help the client move into a more comfortable position.

For a comatose or semicomatose client, you still need to do an introduction. There is no way to know exactly how much a comatose or semicomatose client is taking in. You need to proceed with the assumption that the client can hear and understand what you are saying. Touching someone without any introduction or explanation is frightening, especially if that person has no way to move away from you. For a comatose or semicomatose client, you could begin with the introduction in Box 2-4. Always call the comatose client by his or her last name [**Mr. or Ms. _____**], unless family members insist that the client would prefer to be called by a first name.

STEP 8 Interview the client and/or his or her caregivers.

You need to interview the client to find out who the client is, what his or her interests and priorities are. When the client is unable to speak to you due to illness, coma, confusion, or aphasia, you need to get this information from the client's usual caregivers. Caregivers may include family, friends, and home health aides.

If you do not know clients' priorities, you will not be able to make accurate and realistic discharge recommendations, nor will you be able to effectively collaborate with clients to design meaningful and motivating intervention programs. Appendix A describes some interview assessments that you can use to determine client priorities; the Canadian Occupational Performance Measure (COPM) is especially helpful. Box 2-5 lists some suggested opening questions for a general interview. Figure 2-1, from the occupational therapy evaluation form in Figure 2–29, also provides some guidelines for an initial interview.

An interview is not simply a question and answer session during which the therapist asks questions and records the client's answers. Rather, an interview should be more like a conversation, during which the therapist asks questions that follow-up on what the client has said;

BOX 2-4	INTRODUCTION FOR COMATOSE CLIENT
Hello, I am **[your first and last name]** from occupational therapy. I am here to help you begin moving your arms and legs and begin moving in bed. I'm going to be touching you to help you move.	

BOX 2-5	INITIAL INTERVIEW SUGGESTIONS

- "What brings you to this facility?" **[in inpatient or outpatient settings]** or "What health problems have you been experiencing lately?" **[in home settings].** "How has **[client-identified problem or diagnosis]** affected your day-to-day activities?" "What sorts of things do you need help with now due to your **[client-identified problem or diagnosis]**?" "Has there been any need to change or adapt your home to accommodate your **[client-identified problem or diagnosis]**?"

    The client's answer to these questions will help you to appreciate how the client is understanding and experiencing this current health crisis.

- "Do you live alone?" "In an apartment, a house?" **[for clients with mobility problems],** "Are there stairs to get into your **[apartment or house],** any stairs inside?" "Are there any family or friends who live nearby?" "Are they able to help you out in any way, for example, grocery shopping?"

    The client's answer to these questions will give you an idea about possible barriers and supports after discharge from therapy.

- "Tell me a little about yourself—education, vocational history, marital status, interests and hobbies."

    The client's answer to this question will give you an idea about who this person is and what kind of strengths he or she brings to the therapy process.

- "Tell me about a typical day at home."

    The client's answer to this question will give you some idea about what activities the client considers important and help you to understand the client's usual routines.

- "Which of your day-to-day activities are most important to you?" "Which activities would you most want to do for yourself?" "Which ones would you feel comfortable delegating to someone else?"

    The client's answer to these questions will give you more specific information about the client's activity priorities and about what kinds of changes in his or her usual routine are acceptable to the client.

Note. The questions in this box above are grouped together by general content areas. They are not meant to be asked one question after another. Rather, successive questions are suggested as logical follow-up questions to keep the conversation flowing and provide information about the client.

FIGURE 2-1   Prior Level of Functioning Part of Cedars-Sinai Occupational Therapy Evaluation Profile. Reprinted with permission of Cedars-Sinai Medical Center.

this method of asking questions indicates the therapist has LISTENED carefully to the client. Such careful listening helps establish the rapport so essential to the therapy process.

STEP 9   Observe functional performance and record observations.

Functional activities are often categorized as Basic Activities of Daily Living (BADL) and Instrumental Activities of Daily Living (IADL). Appendix B describes some BADL and IADL assessments. Most times, ADL will be the place you start with functional evaluation. In some outpatient settings, you may begin with work assessments. Table 2-10 lists major functional tasks and the settings where you might evaluate them. The functional tasks listed in Table 2-10 are defined in Appendix H: AOTA's Uniform Terminology for Occupational Therapy, 3rd Edition.

If your practice setting does not have formal ADL assessments available for you to use, you can begin with observation to determine the level of assistance a client needs to complete self-care and mobility tasks. Table 2-11 defines terminology commonly used to describe the levels of assistance a client might need.

You must also use observation to supplement assessments, to provide information on (a) how clients do tasks, (b) how their performance is affected by environmental demands on their sensory processing capacities, and (c) what kinds of compensations clients use in attempting functional tasks. The kinds of errors clients make in ADL and the kinds of successes they have can suggest underlying component skill deficits and strengths, respectively. Table 2-12 provides a structure for your observations. Figures 2-2 through 2-6 can further guide your observations. Figures 2-7 through 2-9 illustrate how your observations of clients performing functional tasks can be used to hypothesize component skill deficits.

With formal assessments of functional activity performance, you will have a specific form to fill out with the rating scale for that assessment, such as the one in Figure 2-10.

If you do not use an assessment, your facility may have specific forms you will need to fill out regarding BADL and IADL status. Figure 2-11, from the occupational therapy evaluation form in Figure 2-29, shows a sample form for recording information about a client's BADL and IADL status.

In some cases, you will need to write a narrative report about the client's functional abilities. For this type of report, you can list the ADL

(text continues on page 41)

TABLE 2-10 | FUNCTIONAL ACTIVITIES TO OBSERVE IN DIFFERENT SETTINGS

Functional Activity	Intensive Care	Acute Care	Inpatient Rehabilitation	Skilled Nursing Facility	Outpatient Rehabilitation
Mobility:					
Bed mobility	•	•	•	•	
Transfers	•	•	•	•	•
Functional ambulation		•	•	•	•
Self-care:					
Feeding & eating	•	•	•	•	
Oral hygiene	•	•	•	•	
Toilet hygiene		•	•	•	
Bathing		•	•	•	
Personal device cleaning		•	•	•	•
Grooming		•	•	•	•
Dressing		•	•	•	•
Medication routine			•	•	•

Homemaking:				
Meal preparation & cleanup		⋅	⋅	⋅
Shopping		⋅	⋅	⋅
Clothing care		⋅	⋅	⋅
Cleaning		⋅	⋅	⋅
Money management		⋅	⋅	⋅
Household maintenance				
Educational activities		⋅	⋅	⋅
Vocational activities			⋅	⋅
Leisure activities			⋅	⋅

Note. See Appendix H for definitions of functional tasks; Mobility & Self-care=Basic Activities of Daily Living (BADL); Homemaking, Educational, Vocational, & Leisure Activities=Instrumental Activities of Daily Living (IADL).

TABLE 2-11	LEVELS OF ASSISTANCE

Level of Assistance	Abbreviation	Definition
Assistive technology	None	Client needs assistive devices like a wheelchair, walker, or long handled reacher to complete BADL tasks
Nonphysical assistance:		
Task set-up	None	Therapist prepares tasks materials and environment for client
Supervision	S	Therapist intermittently checks on client performance and intervenes if needed
Stand-by assistance	SBA	Therapist is in room close to client during BADL performance, intervening as needed
Verbal cues	VC	Therapist gives client oral or written instructions about BADL
Nonverbal cues	None	Therapist uses demonstration and gesture to give client instructions about BADL
Physical assistance:		
Hand-over-hand physical guidance	HOH	Therapist provides hand over hand guidance to get client started
Minimal physical assist	Min A	Therapist assists with 25% of BADL tasks
Moderate physical assist	Mod A	Therapist assists with 50% of BADL tasks
Maximal physical assist	Max A	Therapist assists with 75% of BADL tasks
Dependent	Dep	Therapist assists with more than 75% of BADL tasks or needs to complete task for client

Derived from: Rogers & Holm (1998) and Trombly & Quintana (1989).
Note. BADL = Basic Activities of Daily Living.

| TABLE 2-12 | STRUCTURED OBSERVATION OF ACTIVITIES OF DAILY LIVING PERFORMANCE |

Activity	Performance Errors and Successes	Environmental Demands	Possible Component Skill Deficits	Possible Intervention Strategies
	Errors:	(Noise and lighting levels, number of people client needs to interact with during Activities of Daily Living session, types and arrangement of clothing and toiletries)	Sensory:	(Adapt task method, objects, or environment to capitalize on client's component skill strengths.)
			Perceptual:	
			Cognitive:	
			Motor:	
	Successes:		Psychosocial:	

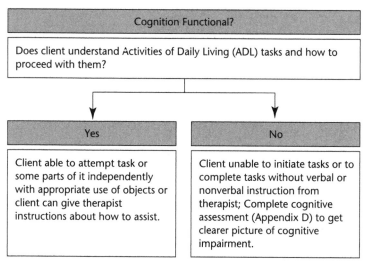

Cognition Functional?

Does client understand Activities of Daily Living (ADL) tasks and how to proceed with them?

Yes	No
Client able to attempt task or some parts of it independently with appropriate use of objects or client can give therapist instructions about how to assist.	Client unable to initiate tasks or to complete tasks without verbal or nonverbal instruction from therapist; Complete cognitive assessment (Appendix D) to get clearer picture of cognitive impairment.

FIGURE 2-2　Guide to Functional Observation of Component Skills/ Cognition

CHAPTER 2

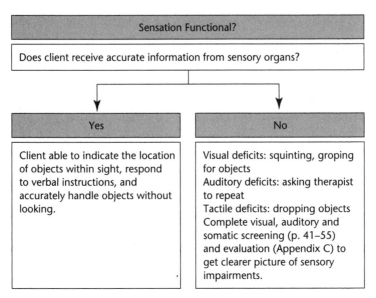

FIGURE 2-3 Guide to Functional Observation of Component Skills/Sensation

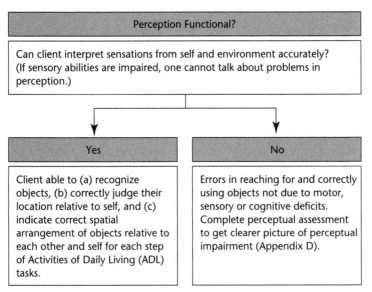

FIGURE 2-4 Guide to Functional Observation of Component Skills/Perception

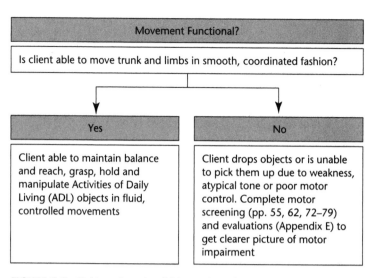

FIGURE 2-5   Guide to Functional Observation of Component Skills/ Movement

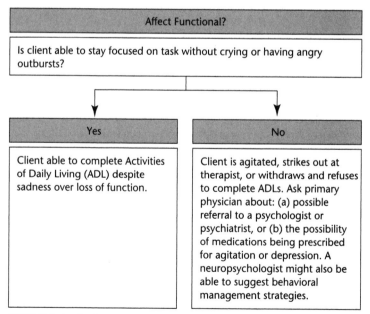

FIGURE 2-6   Guide to Functional Observation of Component Skills/Affect

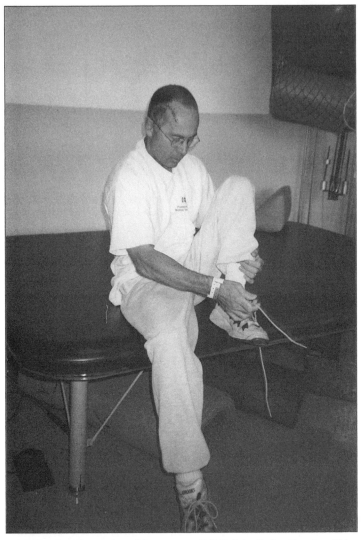

FIGURE 2-7 Observation of Component Skill Deficits During Dressing. This client is using his left hand to help hold his left leg on the mat—a possible indication of decreased strength or motor control in his left leg. He has chosen a method that does not require bending over, raising a question about his balance when he does bend over. Also, given the location of the scar on his head, I would be alert to possible indications of visual field deficits. (Photo courtesy of Cedars-Sinai Medical Center Occupational Therapy Department.)

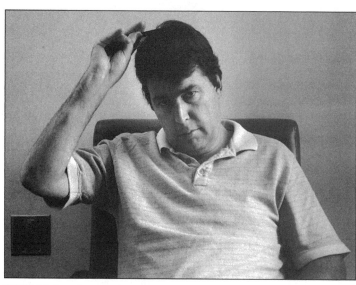

FIGURE 2-8   Observation of Component Skill Deficits During Grooming. This client is bending his head down to meet the comb in his right hand, possibly indicating difficulties with strength or range of motion in his right shoulder. The way he is holding the comb might suggest problems with tone or motor control in the right arm and hand. (Photo courtesy of Cedars-Sinai Medical Center Occupational Therapy Department.)

tasks you evaluated and note the amount of assistance the client needed for each task. You could also note the difficulties you observed with specific component skills. Box 2-6 provides an example of this type of report.

STEP 10   Evaluate component skills contributing to functional performance problems and record evaluation results.

For component skill testing, you should collaborate with other disciplines and avoid duplicate testing. Third-party payers will not pay for duplicate testing. The sequence of component skill testing suggested here is sensory, cognitive/perceptual, motor, psychosocial because motor behaviors can be affected by sensory and cognitive/perceptual deficits.

SENSORY SKILLS

A quick sensory screen should include tests for vision, hearing, and somatic (light touch, deep pressure, pain and temperature, propriocep-

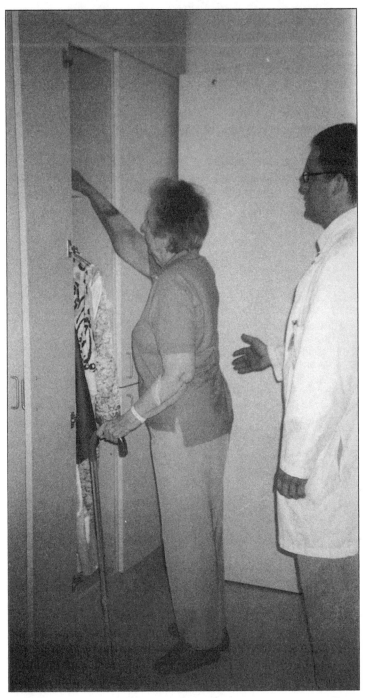

FIGURE 2-9 Observation of Component Skill Deficits During Homemaking. This client needs close guarding to reach into her closet, possibly indicating difficulties with dynamic standing balance. (Photo courtesy of Cedars-Sinai Medical Center Occupational Therapy Department.)

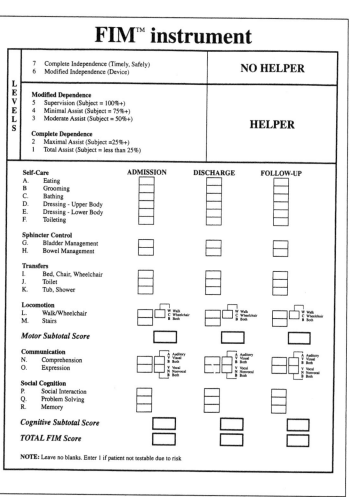

FIGURE 2-10 *Functional Independence Measure* Form. Copyright © 1997 Uniform Data System for Medical Rehabilitation, a division of UB Foundation Activities, Inc. All rights reserved. Reprinted with permission of USDSMR, University at Buffalo, 232 Parker Hall, 3435 Main Street, Buffalo, NY 14214.

tion, kinesthesia) sensation. Tables 2-13 through 2-15 summarize visual, auditory, and somatic sensation screening and reporting procedures. Figures 2-12 through 2-15 illustrate part of the sensory screening procedures for light touch. Figure 2-16, from the occupational therapy evaluation form in Figure 2-29, shows a sample form for recording information about a client's somatic sensory status. Appendix C contains detailed instructions for somatic sensory testing.

Functional Independent Measures (FIMS)			
7 = Independent	CR = Crutches	UE = Upper Extremity	
6 = Modified Independent	NWB = Non Weight Bearing	LE = Lower Extremity	
5 = Supervised/Set-Up	PWB = Partial Weight Bearing	UB = Upper Body	
4 = Min Contact Assist	FWB = Full Weight Bearing	LB = Lower Body	
3 = Moderate Assist		PUW = Pick-Up Walker	
2 = Maximal Assist	LOA = Level of Assist	FWW = Front-Wheel Walker	
1 = Total Assist		SPC = Single Point Cane	
Ref = Patient Refused	NT = Not Tested	W/C = Wheelchair	
		QC = Quadcane	

CODES —

ADL EVALUATION	INTACT	IMPAIRED	COMMENTS / PERFORMANCE COMPONENTS IMPACTING FUNCTION
SWALLOWING			
ORAL PHASE			
PHARYNGEAL PHASE			
DIET			
SELF CARE	ASSIST LEVEL		
FEEDING			
DRESSING - UB			
DRESSING - LB			
GROOMING			
HYGIENE: ORAL			
BATHING			
TOILETING			
FUNCTIONAL MOBILITY	ASSIST LEVEL		
BED			
CHAIR / COUCH			
TOILET TRANSFERS			
TUB/ SHOWER TRANSFERS			
HOME MANAGEMENT			
WORK			
PLAY / LEISURE			

FIGURE 2-11   Codes Box and ADL Evaluation Box From Cedars-Sinai Occupational Therapy Evaluation Profile. Reprinted with permission of Cedars-Sinai Medical Center.

For visual screening, ensure the client is wearing eyeglasses if he or she usually does so. Also, make sure the glasses are clean. Figures 2-17 through 2-20 illustrate screening procedures for a client's visual tracking and visual fields. For auditory screening, if the client uses a hearing aid, make sure he or she is wearing it and that the hearing aide is turned on.

BOX 2-6	SAMPLE NARRATIVE ADL EVALUATION NOTE

Client is a 78-year-old, single woman admitted on 1/30/99 with a diagnosis of left hip fracture and ORIF. She has secondary diagnoses of DJD and HTN. Past medical history includes a possible MI. Client lives alone in an apt with two steps to enter. She is retired from Western Electric. Prior to her hip fracture, she was totally independent in all BADL and IADL. Her priority activities include driving and line dancing. Client is alert, energetic, and motivated to return home. Her BADL status, evaluated on 1/31/99, is as follows:

SELF-CARE

Feeding and eating:	Requires set-up owing to decreased mobility and DJD (opening containers)
Oral hygiene:	Requires only set-up owing to decreased mobility
Toilet hygiene:	Min. A for toilet transfers, Mod. A for managing clothing
Bathing:	Mod. A, with help needed for LEs
Grooming:	Requires only set-up owing to decreased mobility
Dressing:	Min. A for UE dressing, Mod. A for LE dressing
Mobility:	
Bed mobility:	I rolling, Min. A for supine to bed edge
Transfers:	Min. A for all transfers

Client demonstrated functional endurance for self-care. Her difficulties with self-care relate mainly to her postsurgical pain and limited movement of her left hip and partial weight-bearing on left leg. Her DJD also presents her with some difficulties with fine motor aspects of tasks. Her sensation, perception, and cognition are functional for BADL.

Note. ORIF = open reduction, internal fixation; DJD = degenerative joint disease; HTN = hypertension; MI = myocardial infarction; apt = apartment; BADL = Basic Activities of Daily Living (self-care); IADL = Instrumental Activities of Daily Living (community skills); I = independent; Min. = minimal; Mod. = moderate; A = assist; UE = upper extremity; LE = lower extremity.

You should conduct a more complete evaluation of somatic sensation if your screening indicates impairments and for all clients with neurologic diagnoses. For complete evaluation of visual deficits, you may want to recommend a referral to an ophthalmologist or neuroophthalmologist. For complete evaluation of auditory deficits, you may want to recommend a referral to an audiologist.

(text continues on page 55)

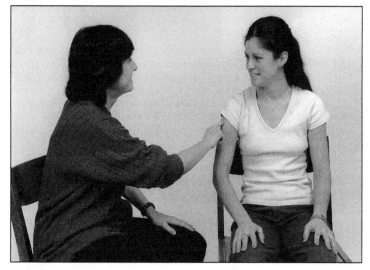

FIGURE 2-12 Light Touch Screening. To screen for differences in proximal to distal sensation in the arms, client is being asked if proximal touch feels the same as distal touch. Photo illustrates proximal touch. (Photos by Ron Bergeron, Instructional Services, Dimond Library, University of New Hampshire, Durham, NH 03824.)

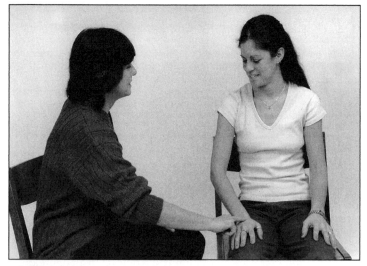

FIGURE 2-13 Light Touch Screening. To screen for differences in proximal to distal sensation in the arms, client is being asked if proximal touch feels the same as distal touch. Photo illustrates distal touch. (Photos by Ron Bergeron, Instructional Services, Dimond Library, University of New Hampshire, Durham, NH 03824.)

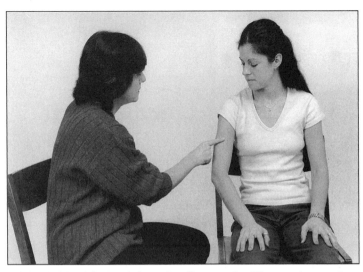

FIGURE 2-14   Light Touch Screening. To screen for differences in sensation between the two arms, client is being asked if right touch feels the same as left touch. Photo illustrates right touch. (Photos by Ron Bergeron, Instructional Services, Dimond Library, University of New Hampshire, Durham, NH 03824.)

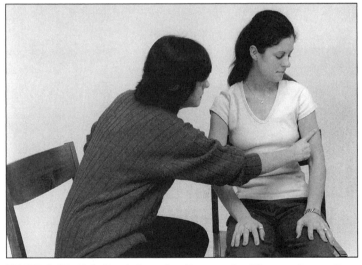

FIGURE 2-15   Light Touch Screening. To screen for differences in sensation between the two arms, client is being asked if right touch feels the same as left touch. Photo illustrates left touch. (Photos by Ron Bergeron, Instructional Services, Dimond Library, University of New Hampshire, Durham, NH 03824.)

SENSORY	INTACT	IMPAIRED	ABSENT
LIGHT TOUCH			
DEEP PRESSURE			
SHARP / DULL			
PROPRIOCEPTION			
KINESTHESIA			
STEREOGNOSIS			

FIGURE 2-16   Sensory Box From Cedars-Sinai Occupational Therapy Evaluation Profile. Reprinted with permission of Cedars-Sinai Medical Center.

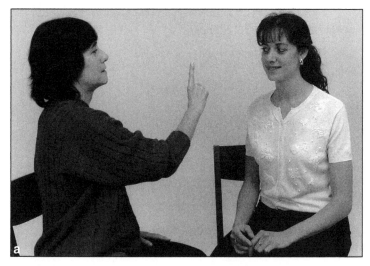

FIGURE 2-17 (a–c)   Visual Tracking Evaluation. To check horizontal tracking, client is being asked to keep her head still and use her eyes to follow the therapist's finger continuously from (a) far left, to (b) midline, to (c) far right. (Photos by Ron Bergeron, Instructional Services, Dimond Library, University of New Hampshire, Durham, NH 03824.)

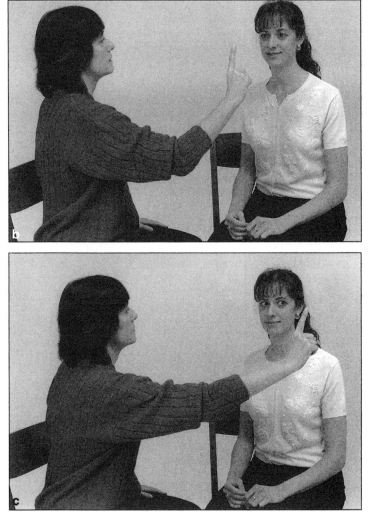

FIGURE 2-17 (a–c)—(*continued*)

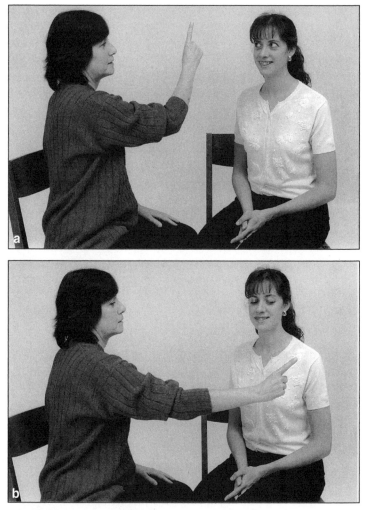

FIGURE 2-18 (a, b)   Visual Tracking Evaluation. To check oblique tracking, client is being asked to keep her head still and use her eyes to follow the therapist's finger continuously from (a) top left, to (b) bottom right. (Photos by Ron Bergeron, Instructional Services, Dimond Library, University of New Hampshire, Durham, NH 03824.)

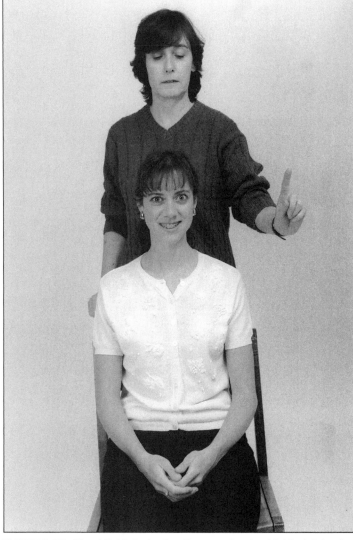

FIGURE 2-19 Visual Fields Evaluation. To screen for visual fields deficits, the therapist moves one finger forward from behind the client's head. The client is asked to say when she first sees the therapist's finger. Photo shows testing of client's left visual field. (Photos by Ron Bergeron, Instructional Services, Dimond Library, University of New Hampshire, Durham, NH 03824.)

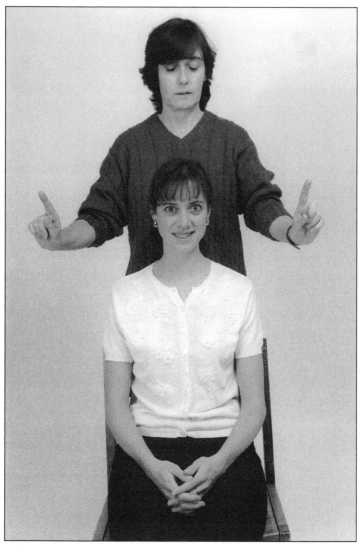

FIGURE 2-20   Visual Fields Evaluation. To screen for visuospatial inattention, the therapist moves two fingers forward from behind the client's head, simultaneously. The client is asked to say when she first sees the therapist's fingers. (Photos by Ron Bergeron, Instructional Services, Dimond Library, University of New Hampshire, Durham, NH 03824.)

CHAPTER 2

TABLE 2-13	VISUAL SCREENING AND REPORTING	
Visual Skill	**Test**	**Sample Reporting of Deficits**
Visual acuity	Distance vision: Functionally, determine client's ability to read far signs (if verbal) or identify far objects by matching (if nonverbal) Near vision: Functionally, determine client's ability to read near signs, greeting cards (if verbal) or identify near objects by matching (if nonverbal)	With eyeglasses can read overhead exit signs _____ feet away, but cannot read a newspaper.
Visual fields	Method one: Confrontation test with two fingers. Stand in front of client, hold your arms out to your sides, elbows bent, hands fisted except for index fingers which are held up straight. Holding your hands first in the upper visual field quadrants, then in the lower quadrants, wiggle first one index finger, then the other, then both, asking client to point to the moving finger. Missing a single wiggling finger indicates a field cut in that quadrant of the visual field. Identifying single wiggling fingers, but missing one side when both fingers are moving indicates visuospatial inattention. Method two: Stand behind client, with your hands fisted except for index fingers which are held up straight. Bring your index fingers forward beside the client's head at ear level, first on one side, then the other. Then bring both hands forward simultaneously. Ask client to tell you when he or she sees a finger. Missing one finger presented alone indicates a field cut on that side. Identifying singly presented fingers, but missing one side when both fingers are presently simultaneously indicates visuospatial inattention.	Client has field cut in [left upper quadrant; entire left side; left lower quadrant] of visual field.
Visual tracking	Have client follow your finger across the visual fields from left to right, then straight up and down, and diagonally (right to left and left to right) to elicit all eye movements.	Client unable to track visual stimuli [horizontally; vertically; diagonally] across visual fields.
Saccadic eye	Have client look quickly from one object to another. Objects should be 6 inches apart and 12–15 inches from client. Only large errors in under or overshooting visual target should be considered abnormal (Bouska Test cited in Zoltan, 1996)	Client unable to shift visual focus quickly from one object to another.

TABLE 2-14 | AUDITORY SCREENING AND REPORTING

Auditory Skill	Test	Sample Reporting
Auditory acuity	While you are speaking to the client, make note of whether he or she needs you to repeat yourself often. Also notice the voice volume that seems to work best for the client.	Client demonstrates difficulty hearing normal voice volume.
Ability to separate one voice or sound from background noise	Note whether client has difficulty engaging in conversation with you with background noise (public address system, television, radio, other people in room talking) compared to client's ability to converse with you in a quiet setting.	Client is unable to screen out extraneous noise to focus on a particular sound or speaker.
Auditory processing	Note quickness of client's response when you speak rapidly versus slowly. (Difficulty responding when you speak rapidly may indicate slowed auditory processing.)	Client is slow to respond to rapid speech, but responds well to slowed speech.

TABLE 2-15	SOMATIC SENSORY SCREENING AND REPORTING

Somatic Sensory Skill	Test	Sample Reporting of Deficits
General somatic sensory acuity and quality	Ask client, "Do you have any problems with numbness or pins & needles in your arms or hands?"	Client reports [constant, intermittent] pins and needles sensations in right hand; sensations more pronounced [at time of day; during _____ activity].
Light touch sensation along peripheral nerve distributions	Touch the client lightly from proximal to distal on each arm and ask, "Does this feel the same all the way down your arm?" (screen for peripheral neuropathy)	Client's light touch sensation impaired below [elbows; wrists] on both UEs.
Cortical perception of light touch	Touch the client lightly on one arm, then the other and ask, "Does this feel the same on both sides of your body?" (screen for lesion in cortical sensory strip)	Client's light touch sensation impaired on [L,R]UE, WNL on [L,R]UE.

Note. UE = upper extremity; L = left; R = right; WNL = within normal limits.

COGNITIVE/PERCEPTUAL SKILLS

Table 2-16 will help you identify specific cognitive/perceptual deficits during observations of clients' BADLs and IADLs. Figure 2-21 will help you identify patterns of cognitive function for adults with traumatic brain injury. Figure 2-22, from the occupational therapy evaluation form in Figure 2-29, shows a sample form for recording information about clients' perceptual and cognitive abilities. See Appendix D for a description of cognitive/perceptual assessments.

MOTOR SKILLS

A quick way to evaluate upper extremity active range of motion (AROM) is pictured in Figures 2-23 through 2-25. See Appendix E for a description of motor assessments and formal procedures for motor
(text continues on page 62)

TABLE 2-16	PERCEPTUAL/COGNITIVE SKILLS AND DEFICITS AND REPORTING	

Skill or Deficit	Definition	Examples of Functional Problems
VISUAL SKILLS Visual attention	Voluntary act of visual fixation; focused gaze Visual spatial inattention: Decreased awareness of body and spatial environment on side contralateral to cerebral lesion despite the absence of a specific sensory deficit, with or without visual field deficits	Persons without this skill might have trouble reading, watching television, maintaining eye contact during conversation, or any activity that requires visual focusing
APRAXIA Constructional apraxia	Inability to put parts of things together into a whole	Persons with this deficit would have problems setting a table, copying a drawing from the blackboard, making a sandwich
Motor apraxia	Loss of kinesthetic memory patterns (brain programs for different types of movements)	Persons with this deficit would have difficulty doing any activity even though they would know what they wanted to do
Ideomotor apraxia	Inability to imitate gestures or carry out purposeful movements on command while retaining the ability to perform routine, automatic activities	Persons with this deficit would have problems following an aerobic class or learning a new craft activity
Ideational apraxia	Inability to carry out routine activities because the person does not understand the concept of the activity	Persons with this deficit would have problems with all activities
BODY SCHEME Somatognosia	Unawareness of body structure and failure to recognize one's body parts and their relation to each other	Persons with this deficit would have difficulty learning a new sport, learning how to use a wheelchair or walker, or how to do transfers

Common Lesion Sites	Sample Reporting of Deficits
Frontal lobes: body centered inattention Parietal lobes: environment centered inattention Usually right hemisphere	Client has difficulty focusing visual attention during functional activities.
Bilateral brain lesions; lesions to either cortical hemisphere; inferior parietal association area; posterior hemispheric lesions; frontal lobe lesions; corpus callosal lesions; subcortical lesions; diffuse brain injury	Client demonstrates constructional deficits, i.e., difficulty with functional tasks requiring assembly like [task you saw client have problems with]
Frontal lobe, premotor cortex, either hemisphere	Client has difficulty planning movements during functional tasks.
Parietal lobe, supramarginal gyrus, dominant hemisphere; left frontal lobe; premotor cortex	Client has difficulty planning movements during functional tasks.
Inferior parietal association area of dominant hemisphere; diffuse brain injury; orbitofrontal or dorsolateral frontal areas; premotor cortex	Client has difficulty planning movements during functional tasks.
Inferior parietal association cortex, dominant hemisphere	Client demonstrates difficulty knowing how to move body during functional tasks.

continued

CHAPTER 2

TABLE 2-16	PERCEPTUAL/COGNITIVE SKILLS AND DEFICITS AND REPORTING (CONTINUED)

Skill or Deficit	Definition	Examples of Functional Problems
Finger agnosia	Inability to consistently name the fingers	Persons with this deficit would have difficulty following instructions for finger exercises
Right-left discrimination	Ability to tell left from right on oneself and in the environment	Persons without this skill would have difficulty following directions about how to get from one place to another
VISUAL DISCRIMINATION Figure ground	Ability to distinguish the foreground from the background	Persons without this skill would have problems picking a kitchen utensil out of a cluttered drawer or seeing variations in terrain while walking
Form constancy	Ability to recognize an object as being the same when seen from different views	Persons without this skill would have difficulty telling the difference between street signs
Depth perception (stereopsis)	Ability to perceive three dimensional space	Persons without this skill would have difficulty parking a car or judging the height of stairs
Spatial relations	Ability to perceive self in relation to other objects	Persons without this skill would have difficulty with moving in new environments or accurately reaching for objects
Detail and contour discrimination	Ability to accurately perceive both the details and the contours of objects	Persons who focus on details might have difficulty using the telephone due to distraction with the buttons and numbers Persons who focus on the contour might have difficulty discriminating between products with similar packaging in the grocery store

Common Lesion Sites	Sample Reporting of Deficits
Parietal lobe, angular gyrus, either hemisphere	Client unable to consistently name his/her fingers
Inferior parietal association cortex, either hemisphere	Client unable to tell left from right during functional tasks.
Inferior parietal association cortex, non-dominant hemisphere; large lesion or small lesions anywhere in brain	Client unable to distinguish the foreground from the background during functional tasks.
Inferior parietal association cortex, non-dominant hemisphere	Client unable to recognize objects from different views during functional tasks.
Visual cortices	Client demonstrating depth perception deficits functionally.
Inferior parietal association cortex, non-dominant hemisphere	Client demonstrating spatial relations deficits functionally.
Nondominant hemisphere: derive information from the details	Client unable to accurately perceive both the details and the contours of functional objects.
Dominant hemisphere: derive information from the contours	

continued

TABLE 2-16	PERCEPTUAL/COGNITIVE SKILLS AND DEFICITS AND REPORTING (CONTINUED)

Skill or Deficit	Definition	Examples of Functional Problems
AGNOSIA		
Visual object agnosia	Inability to recognize objects	Persons with this deficit would have trouble finding their coats in a coat room or their cars in a parking lot
Prosopagnosia	Inability to recognize faces	Persons with this deficit would have difficulty recognizing people they have met
Simultagnosia	Inability to synthesize multiple visual stimuli	Persons with this deficit would have difficulty reading (seeing letters as part of a whole word), working complex machinery
COGNITIVE SKILLS		
Orientation ×3	Awareness of time, person, and place	Persons without this skill would: not answer to their own names; not know the time of day, date or season; and get lost easily
Attention	Ability to focus on particular sensory stimuli	Persons without this skill would be distractible and have difficulty completing tasks
Memory	Ability to recall or recognize information or procedures	Persons without this skill would lose track of what they were doing, have difficulty completing tasks, or keeping appointments
Initiation	Ability to begin a task in a timely fashion	Persons without this skill would not begin daily tasks without cuing
Self-monitoring/awareness	Ability to accurately anticipate one's performance potentials and judge the adequacy of actual task performance	Persons without this skill might engage in unsafe behavior due to lack of awareness about performance limitations
Planning, organization, and sequencing	Ability to map out a logical, step by step, approach to multiple tasks	Persons without this skill might be very disorganized and scattered and have difficulty getting things done on time
		Persons with severe sequencing deficits may demonstrate perseveration

Common Lesion Sites	Sample Reporting of Deficits
Inferior parietal association cortex, non-dominant hemisphere	Client unable to recognize functional objects.
Inferior occipital lobes, bilaterally	Client unable to recognize [new; familiar] faces.
Occipital-parietal lobe, dominant hemisphere	Client has difficulty synthesizing multiple visual stimuli during functional tasks.
Nondominant parietal lobe: topographical orientation	Client disoriented to [time; person; place or ×3 if disoriented to all of these]
Brain stem reticular activating system, limbic lobes, prefrontal dorsolateral cortex	Client is very distractible and has difficulty completing functional tasks.
Temporal lobe, limbic lobe, orbitofrontal area, generalized throughout brain	Client has difficulty with memory during functional tasks.
Frontal lobes, orbitofrontal areas	Client needs cues to initiate functional tasks.
Pre-frontal cortex: poor awareness of social skills and poor ability to anticipate change Parietal lobes: Poor awareness of body image, and of sensory, perceptual, and motor abilities	Client unable to accurately judge own abilities.
Frontal lobes	Client has difficulty with planning, sequencing, and organizing functional tasks.

continued

TABLE 2-16	PERCEPTUAL/COGNITIVE SKILLS AND DEFICITS AND REPORTING (CONTINUED)

Skill or Deficit	Definition	Examples of Functional Problems
Problem solving	Ability to identify difficulties in task performance and generate viable solutions	Persons without this skill would not know what to do in difficult situations, eg, a water heater leak
Mental flexibility and abstraction	Ability to conceptualize multiple perspectives and task approaches	Persons without this skill would be unable to adjust to unexpected changes in daily routines
Calculation	Ability to manipulate numbers	Persons without this skill would be unable to manage own finances
Time perception	Ability to accurately perceive the passage of time	Persons without this skill would not be punctual in keeping appointments

Derived from: Årnadøttir (1990); Neistadt (1994); Scheiman (1997); Zoltan (1996); Zoltan, Siev, & Freishtat (1986).

testing. Figure 2-26 will help you decide how to proceed after this AROM screening.

Table 2-17 delineates additional motor screening procedures. All of the tests in this table would be appropriate for clients who show impairments in the range or quality of their AROM; the strength, endurance, coordination, and balance tests would be appropriate for clients with full AROM with good quality movement.

Table 2-18 provides definitions of types of atypical muscle tone you might feel in clients with neurologic diagnoses. Table 2-19 defines categories of spasticity.

Muscles with atypical tone should not be tested for strength because you cannot accurately assess strength in these muscles. If manual muscle testing is needed, you should perform this testing only on those muscles in which clients have normal tone. Table 2-20 lists grading systems for manual muscle testing. Figure 2-27, from the occupational therapy evaluation form in Figure 2–29, shows a sample form for recording information about clients' motor skills.

Common Lesion Sites	Sample Reporting of Deficits
Frontal lobes	Client has difficulty with problem solving functionally.
Frontal lobes	Client has difficulty with mental flexibility & abstraction functionally.
Dominant occipital lobe: acalculia Dominant partial lobe: discalculia	Client has difficulty with calculation functionally.
Nondominant hemisphere: time perceived as passing quickly and client may be impulsive Dominant hemisphere: time is perceived as passing slowly	Client has difficulty with time perception functionally.

PSYCHOSOCIAL SKILLS

All clients are referred to you because they have experienced a loss of function that has disrupted their lives. Consequently, all clients will feel distressed to some degree. Those with physical illness or injury may be in pain, upset about issues of body image, or frustrated by their limited ability to move around and do things for themselves. Those with brain dysfunction, whether from stroke or mental illness, may be confused and feel frightened as a result. You need to be aware of the emotional comfort of all clients, as well as the effects of those comfort levels on functional performance.

For clients with mental illness, the main aim of your evaluation is to determine how their psychosocial problems affect their BADL and IADL performance. Appendix F describes some assessments that have been developed to achieve that purpose with this client group. You also need to be alert with these clients to physical problems stemming from psychotropic medication side effects.

(text continues on page 82)

Rancho Levels of Cognitive Functioning - Revised

Patient Name: _____ Diagnosis: _____

MR#: _____ Date of Onset: _____

Level of Function	Behavioral Characteristics	Examiners						
		Assessment Dates						
Level 1 No Response Total Assistance	• Complete absence of observable change in behavior when presented visual, auditory, tactile, proprioceptive, vestibular or painful stimuli.							
Level 2 Generalized Response	• Demonstrates generalized reflex response to painful stimuli.							
	• Responds to repeated auditory stimuli with increased or decreased activity.							
Total Assistance	• Responds to external stimuli with physiological changes generalized, gross body movement and /or not purposeful vocalization.							
	Responses noted above may be same regardless of type and location of stimulation.							
	Responses may be significantly delayed.							
Level 3 Localized Response	Demonstrates withdrawal or vocalization to painful stimili.							
	• Turns toward or away from auditory stimuli.							
	• Blinks when strong light crosses visual field.							
Total Assistance	• Follows moving object passed within visual field.							
	• Responds to discomfort by pulling tubes or restraints.							
	• Responds inconsistently to simple commands.							
	• Responses directly related to type of stimulus.							
	• May respond to some persons (especially family and friends) but not to others.							

FIGURE 2-21   Rancho Levels of Cognitive Functioning. Assessment form for *Rancho Levels of Cognitive Functioning. A Clinical Case Management Tool,* 3rd ed., © 1998, Chris Hagen, PhD, CCC-SLP. Reprinted with permission from Dr. Hagen, 908 Via Linda, Escondido, CA 92029.

Level of Function	Behavioral Characteristics	Examiners						
		Assessment Dates						
Level 4	• Alert and in heightened state of activity							
Confused-Agitated	• Purposeful attempts to remove restraints or tubes or crawl out of bed.							
Maximal Assistance	• May perform motor activities such as sitting, reaching and walking but without any apparent purpose or upon another's request.							
	• Very brief and usually non purposeful moments of sustained alternatives and divided attention.							
	• Absent short-term memory.							
	• Absent goal directed, problem solving, self-monitoring behavior.							
	• May cry out or scream out of proportion to stimulus even after its removal.							
	• May exhibit aggressive or flight behavior.							
	Mood may swing from euphoric to hostile with no apparent relationship to environmental events.							
	• Unable to cooperate with treatment efforts.							
	• Verbalizations are frequently incoherent and/or inappropriate to activity or environment.							
Level 5	• Alert, not agitated but may wander randomly or with a vague intention of going home.							
Confused - Inappropriate - Non-Agitated	• May become agitated in response to external stimulation and/or lack of environmental structure.							
	• Not oriented to person, place or time.							
Maximal Assistance	• Frequent brief periods, non-purposeful sustained attention.							
	• Severely impaired recent memory, with confusion of past and present in reaction to ongoing activity.							
	• Absent goal-directed, problem-solving, self-monitoring behavior							

FIGURE 2-21—(continued)

Level of Function	Behavioral Characteristics	Examiners					
		Assessment Dates					
Level 5 Continued	• Often demonstrates inappropriate use of objects without external direction.						
	• May be able to perform previously learned tasks when structure and cues provided.						
	• Unable to learn new information.						
	• Able to respond appropriately to simple commands fairly consistently with external structures and cues.						
	• Responses to simple commands without external structure are random and non-purposeful in relation to the command.						
	• Able to converse on a social, automatic level for brief periods of time when provided external structure and cues.						
	• Verbalizations about present events become inappropriate and confabulatory when external structure and cues are not provided.						
Level 6 Confused-Appropriate Moderate Assistance	• Inconsistently oriented to person and place						
	• Able to attend to highly familiar tasks in non-distracting environment for 30 minutes with moderate redirection.						
	• Remote memory has more depth and detail than recent memory.						
	• Vague recognition of some staff.						
	• Able to use assistive memory aide with Max assist.						
	• Emerging awareness of appropriate response to self, family and basic needs.						
	• Emerging goal directed behavior related to meeting basic personal needs.						
	• Moderate assist to problem solve barriers to task completion.						
	• Supervised for old learning (e.g., self-care)						
	• Shows carry over for relearned familiar tasks (e.g., self-care)						

FIGURE 2-21—(*continued*)

Level of Function	Behavioral Characteristics	Examiners					
		Assessment Dates					
Level 6 Continued	• Max assist for new learning with little or no carry over.						
	• Unaware of impairments, disabilities and safety risks.						
	• Consistently follows simple directions.						
	• Verbal expressions are appropriate in highly familiar and structured situations						
Level 7 Automatic - Appropriate Minimal Assistance For Routine Daily Living Skills	• Consistently oriented to person and place, within highly familiar environments. Mod. assist for orientation to time.						
	• Able to attend to highly familiar tasks in a nondistraction environment for at least 30 minutes with minimal assist to complete tasks.						
	• Able to use assistive memory devices with Minimal assistance.						
	• Minimal supervision for new learning.						
	• Demonstrates carry over of new learning.						
	• Initiates and carries out steps to complete familiar personal and household routine but has shallow recall of what he/she has been doing.						
	• Able to monitor accuracy and completeness of each step in routine personal and household ADLs and modify plan with minimum assistance.						
	• Superficial awareness of his/her condition but unaware of specific impairments and disabilities and the limits they place on his/her ability to safely, accurately and completely carry out his/her household, community, work and leisure ADLs.						
	• Minimal supervision for safety in routine home and community activities.						
	• Unrealistic planning for the future.						
	• Unable to think about consequences of a decision or action.						
	• Overestimate abilities.						

FIGURE 2-21—(*continued*)

Level of Function	Behavioral Characteristics	Examiners						
		Assessment Dates						
Level 7 Continued	• Unaware of others' needs and feelings.							
	• Oppositional/uncooperative							
	• Unable to recognize inappropriate social interaction behavior.							
Level 8 Purposeful and Appropriate Stand-by Assistance	• Consistently oriented to person, place and time.							
	• Independently attends to and completes familiar tasks for 1 hour in a distracting environment.							
	• Able to recall and integrate past and recent events.							
	• Uses assistive memory devices to recall daily schedule, "to do" lists and record critical information for later use with stand-by assistance.							
	• Initiates and carries out steps to complete familiar personal, household, community, work and leisure routines with stand-by assistance and can modify the plan when needed with minimal assistance.							
	• Requires no assistance once new tasks/activities are learned.							
	• Aware of and acknowledges impairments and disabilities when they interfere with task completion but requires stand-by assistance to take appropriate corrective action.							
	• Thinks about consequences of a decision or action with minimal assistance.							
	• Overestimates or underestimates abilities.							
	• Acknowledges others' needs and feelings and responds appropriately with minimal assistance.							
	• Depressed.							
	• Irritable.							
	• Low frustration tolerance/easily angered.							
	• Argumentative.							

FIGURE 2-21—(*continued*)

Level of Function	Behavioral Characteristics	Examiners						
		Assessment Dates						
Level 8 Continued	• Self centered.							
	• Uncharacteristically dependent/independent.							
	• Able to recognize and acknowledge inappropriate social interaction behavior while it is occurring and takes corrective action with minimal assistance.							
Level 9 Purposeful and Appropriate	• Independently shifts back and forth between tasks and completes them accurately for at least two consecutive hours.							
Stand-by Assistance on Request	• Uses assistive memory devices to recall daily schedule, "to do" lists and record critical information for later use with assistance when requested.							
	• Initiates and carries out steps to complete familiar personal, household, work and leisure tasks independently and unfamiliar personal, household, work and leisure tasks with assistance when requested.							
	• Aware of and acknowledges impairments and disabilities when they interfere with task completion and takes appropriate corrective action but requires stand-by assist to anticipate a problem before it occurs and take action to avoid it.							
	• Able to think about consequences of decisions or actions with assistance when requested.							
	• Accurately estimates abilities but requires stand-by assistance to adjust to task demands.							
	• Acknowledges others' needs and feelings and responds appropriately with stand-by assistance.							
	• Depression may continue.							
	• May be easily irritable.							
	• May have low frustration tolerance.							
	• Able to self-monitor appropriateness of social interaction with stand-by assist.							

FIGURE 2-21—(continued)

Level of Function	Behavioral Characteristics	Examiners						
		Assessment Dates						
Level 10	• Able to handle multiple tasks simultaneously in all environments but may require periodic breaks.							
Purposeful and Appropriate	• Able to independently procure, create and maintain own assistive memory devices.							
Modified Independent	• Independently initiates and carries out steps to complete familiar and unfamiliar personal, household, community, work and leisure tasks but may require more than the usual amount of time and/or compensatory strategies to complete them.							
	• Anticipates impact of impairments and disabilities on ability to complete daily living tasks and takes action to avoid problems before they occur but may require more than the usual amount of time and/or compensatory strategies.							
	• Able to independently think about consequences of decisions or action but may require more than the usual amount of time and/or compensatory strategies to select the appropriate decision or action.							
	• Accurately estimates abilities and independently adjusts to task demands.							
	• Able to recognize the needs and feelings of others and automatically respond in appropriate manner.							
	• Periodic periods of depression may occur.							
	• Irritability and low frustration tolerance when sick, fatigued, and /or under emotional stress.							
	• Social interaction behavior is consistently appropriate.							

FIGURE 2-21—(continued)

COGNITION

CONSCIOUSNESS ☐ ALERT   ☐ LETHARGIC   ☐ FLUCTUATING
☐ STUPOROUS   ☐ COMATOSE
IF TBI: RANCHO SCALE_____

ORIENTATION: ☐ TIME ☐ PLACE ☐ PERSON ☐ SITUATION

ATTENTION SPAN: _____ SECONDS / MINUTES FOR IMMEDIATE ATTENTION
_____ MINUTES FOR SUSTAINED ATTENTION

	INTACT	IMPAIRED		INTACT	IMPAIRED
SEQUENCING			PROBLEM SOLVING / REASONING		
MEMORY SHORT TERM			JUDGEMENT / SAFETY		
MEMORY LONG TERM					

PERCEPTION	INTACT	IMPAIRED		INTACT	IMPAIRED
VISUAL FIELD			DEPTH PERCEPTION		
VISUAL ATTENTION			MOTOR PLANNING		
R / L DISCRIMINATION					
BODY AWARENESS / SCHEME					

COMMENTS:

FIGURE 2-22 Cognition and Perception Boxes From Cedars-Sinai Occupational Therapy Evaluation Profile. Reprinted with permission of Cedars-Sinai Medical Center.

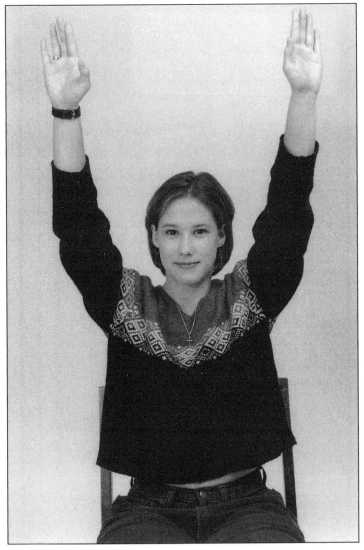

FIGURE 2-23   Active Range of Motion (AROM) Screening. To check for limitations in shoulder flexion, the client is asked to raise her arms overhead as high as she can. (Photos by Ron Bergeron, Instructional Services, Dimond Library, University of New Hampshire, Durham, NH 03824.)

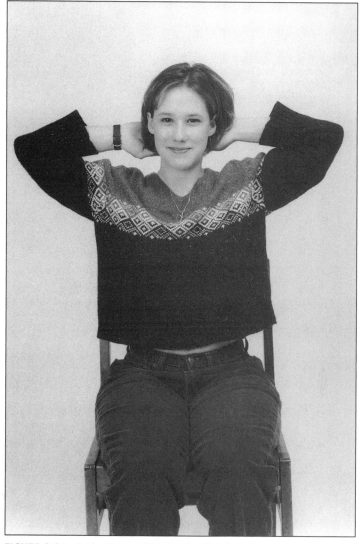

FIGURE 2-24 Active Range of Motion (AROM) Screening. To check for limitations in shoulder external rotation, the client is asked to put her arms behind her neck. (Photos by Ron Bergeron, Instructional Services, Dimond Library, University of New Hampshire, Durham, NH 03824.)

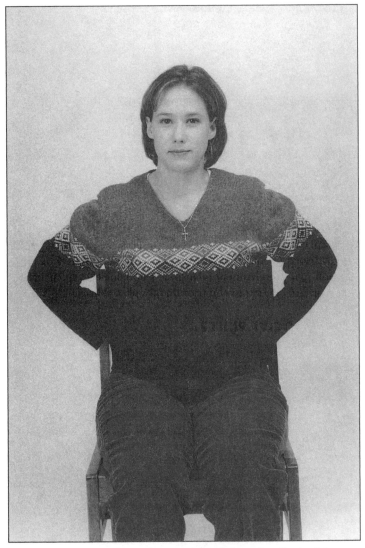

FIGURE 2-25   Active Range of Motion (AROM) Screening. To check for limitations in shoulder internal rotation, the client is asked to put her arms behind her lower back. (Photos by Ron Bergeron, Instructional Services, Dimond Library, University of New Hampshire, Durham, NH 03824.)

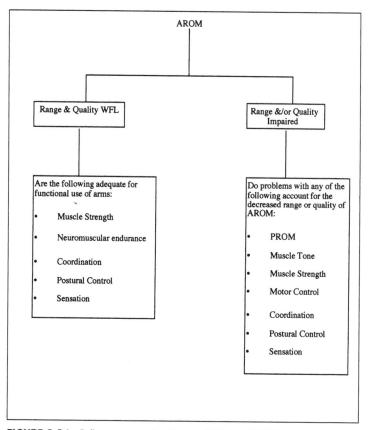

FIGURE 2-26   Follow-up to Active Range of Motion (AROM) Screening
Note. AROM = active range of motion; PROM = passive range of motion;
WFL = within functional limits

TABLE 2-17	MOTOR SCREENING AND REPORTING

Motor Skill	Test	Sample Reporting of Deficits
Joint Flexibility	Passive Range of Motion (PROM) of Upper Extremities (UEs)—feel for muscle tone as you do this.	Client has [1/4;1/2;3/4] range for shoulder [abduction, adduction, internal/external rotation; flexion; extension], elbow [flexion; extension], forearm [supination;pronation], wrist [flexion/ext].
Muscle Tone	Quick stretch of biceps to check for spasticity.	Client has [minimal; moderate; severe] spasticity in [muscle groups or throughout [L;R] UE].
Muscle Strength	Manual Muscle Testing (MMT) of major muscle groups (e.g., shoulder flexors, shoulder abductors, elbow flexors & extensors, mass grasp for finger flexors) with normal tone.	Client has [muscle grade] strength in [muscle groups].
Muscle Endurance	Note client's ability to sustain full available movement throughout the session without complaints of fatigue or decrease in amount and force of movement.	Client only able to sustain full motion for _____ minutes.
Motor Control	If client can move arms, have client touch therapist's index finger (held out in front of client), first with one hand, then the other.	Client's movements are not smooth and well controlled.
Coordination	If client can move hands, have client do rapid supination & pronation with arms stretched out in front. If client can move hands, have client do rapid touching of fingertips to thumb, one at a time, starting with the index finger.	Client has impaired fine motor coordination in [R;L; both [UE(s); hand(s)].
Postural Control	Observe client's ability to maintain sitting balance throughout motor screening.	Client unable to maintain sitting balance during motor screening.

Note. L = left; R = right; UE = upper extremity.

TABLE 2-18	ATYPICAL MUSCLE TONE DEFINITIONS	
Type of Atypical Tone	**Definition**	**Clinical Manifestations**
Hypotonia	Decreased muscle tone resulting from hypo-responsiveness to sensory stimulation	Muscles appear soft, flabby, and lax; passive range of motion may be greater than normal due to lax muscles
Spasticity	Increased muscle tone, especially with quick stretch; tone may "let go" near the end of the range	Muscles appear tight and toned; tight muscles create resistance to passive range of motion
Rigidity	Simultaneous increase of muscle tone in agonist and antagonist muscles resulting in increased resistance to passive range of motion in any direction throughout the range	Lead pipe rigidity—muscles are rigid, arm is hard to move throughout the range Cogwheel rigidity—tremor superimposed on rigidity causing alternate contraction and relaxation throughout the range
Tremors, Choreas, Athetoid Movements, Ballism	Uncontrolled fluctuations of muscle tone in agonist and antagonist muscles	Tremors—Shaky movements that can occur either at rest (resting tremor), with motion (intention tremor), or both Choreas—jerky, irregular, brisk graceful movements of limbs accompanied by involuntary twitching and grimacing of face Athetoid movements—slow writhing movements Ballism—uncontrolled flinging of extremities

CHAPTER 2

Reprinted from: Kohlmeyer, K. (1998). Evaluation of sensory and neuromuscular performance components. In M. E. Neistadt & E. B. Crepeau (Eds.), *Willard & Spackman's occupational therapy,* 9th ed. (pp. 223–260). Philadelphia: Lippincott, p. 233, with permission.

TABLE 2-19 CATEGORIES OF SPASTICITY

Mild Spasticity	Moderate Spasticity	Severe Spasticity
▪ stretch reflex occurs in last 1/4 of range	▪ stretch reflex occurs mid-range	▪ stretch reflex occurs in initial 1/4 range
▪ slight imbalance in tone between agonist and antagonist	▪ marked imbalance of tone between agonist and antagonist	▪ severe imbalance of tone between agonist and antagonist
▪ mild increased resistance to passive stretch	▪ considerable resistance to passive stretch; able to move through full PROM	▪ marked resistance to passive movement, unable to complete full PROM
▪ may exhibit slight decreased mobility and ability to perform fine, selective movements	▪ may exhibit slow gross movements which require increased effort and show decreased coordination	▪ significant decreased or lack of active movement, may exhibit joint contractures

Note. PROM = Passive Range of Motion (Mathiowetz & Haugen, 1995; Undzis, Zoltan, & Pedretti, 1996)
Reprinted from Kohlmeyer, K. (1998). Evaluation of sensory and neuromuscular performance components. In M. E. Neistadt & E. B. Crepeau (Eds.), *Willard & Spackman's occupational therapy,* 9th ed. (pp. 223–260). Philadelphia: Lippincott, p. 235, with permission.

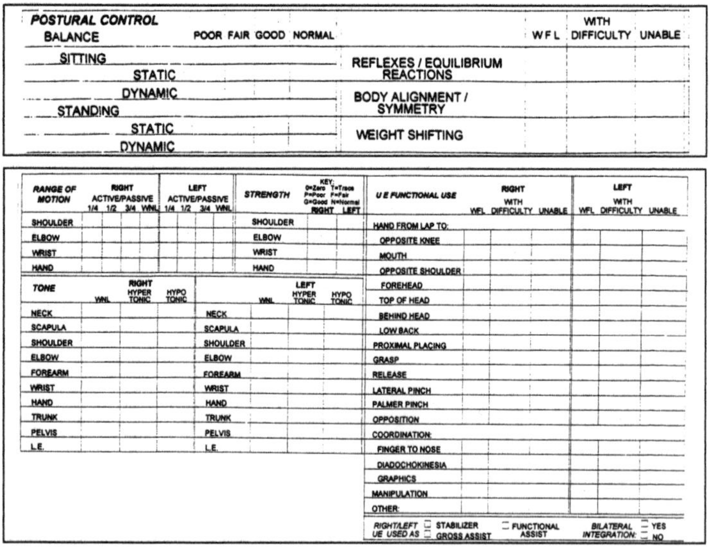

POSTURAL CONTROL BALANCE	POOR	FAIR	GOOD	NORMAL
SITTING				
STATIC				
DYNAMIC				
STANDING				
STATIC				
DYNAMIC				

	WFL	WITH DIFFICULTY	UNABLE
REFLEXES / EQUILIBRIUM REACTIONS			
BODY ALIGNMENT / SYMMETRY			
WEIGHT SHIFTING			

RANGE OF MOTION	RIGHT ACTIVE/PASSIVE 1/4	1/2	3/4	WNL	LEFT ACTIVE/PASSIVE 1/4	1/2	3/4	WNL
SHOULDER								
ELBOW								
WRIST								
HAND								

STRENGTH (KEY: 0=Zero T=Trace P=Poor F=Fair G=Good N=Normal)	RIGHT	LEFT
SHOULDER		
ELBOW		
WRIST		
HAND		

TONE	RIGHT WNL	RIGHT HYPER TONIC	RIGHT HYPO TONIC		LEFT WNL	LEFT HYPER TONIC	LEFT HYPO TONIC
NECK				NECK			
SCAPULA				SCAPULA			
SHOULDER				SHOULDER			
ELBOW				ELBOW			
FOREARM				FOREARM			
WRIST				WRIST			
HAND				HAND			
TRUNK				TRUNK			
PELVIS				PELVIS			
L.E.				L.E.			

U E FUNCTIONAL USE	RIGHT WFL	RIGHT WITH DIFFICULTY	RIGHT UNABLE	LEFT WFL	LEFT WITH DIFFICULTY	LEFT UNABLE
HAND FROM LAP TO:						
OPPOSITE KNEE						
MOUTH						
OPPOSITE SHOULDER						
FOREHEAD						
TOP OF HEAD						
BEHIND HEAD						
LOW BACK						
PROXIMAL PLACING						
GRASP						
RELEASE						
LATERAL PINCH						
PALMER PINCH						
OPPOSITION						
COORDINATION:						
FINGER TO NOSE						
DIADOCHOKINESIA						
GRAPHICS						
MANIPULATION						
OTHER:						

RIGHT/LEFT UE USED AS ☐ STABILIZER ☐ GROSS ASSIST ☐ FUNCTIONAL ASSIST   BILATERAL INTEGRATION: ☐ YES ☐ NO

FIGURE 2-27 Range of Motion, UE Functional Use, Tone, Strength, and Postural Control Boxes From Cedars-Sinai Occupational Therapy Evaluation Profile. Reprinted with permission of Cedars-Sinai Medical Center.

TABLE 2-20	MANUAL MUSCLE TESTING GRADING SYSTEMS

Numerical Scale	Letter Grade	Letter Grade Abbreviation	Definition
5	Normal	N	Able to move part through full ROM against gravity and hold against maximal resistance at end of range
4	Good	G	Able to move part through full ROM against gravity and take moderate resistance at end of range
	Good minus	G−	Able to move part through full ROM against gravity and take less than moderate resistance at end of range
	Fair plus	F+	Able to move part through full ROM against gravity and take minimal resistance at end of range
3	Fair	F	Able to move part through full ROM against gravity, but not able to take any resistance at end of range
	Fair minus	F−	Able to move part through more than one half ROM against gravity
	Poor plus	P+	Able to move part through less than one half ROM against gravity
2	Poor	P	Able to move part through full ROM in gravity-eliminated position
	Poor minus	P−	Able to move part through more than one half ROM in gravity-eliminated position
	Trace plus	T+	Able to move part through less than one half ROM in gravity-eliminated position
1	Trace	T	Contraction can be palpated—no movement
0	Zero	0	No palpable contraction

Note. ROM = range of motion; Compiled from Kohlmeyer (1998) and Trombly & Scott (1989).

CHAPTER 2

TABLE 2-21	OCCUPATIONAL THERAPY APPROACHES FOR DIFFERENT LEVELS OF INFORMATION PROCESSING

Allen Cognitive Disability Level	Learning Characteristics & Cuing Needed	Intervention Approach
Level 0: Coma	The client is unconscious for a prolonged period of time and does not respond to stimuli.	Structure environment to provide sensory stimulation that is meaningful to the client; instruct caregivers on passive range of motion techniques and good body mechanics for moving client.
Level 1: Automatic Actions	The client is conscious and responds to stimuli. He or she is dependent for all self-care tasks, and requires 24-hour supervision	Structure environment, instruct caregivers, on how to best assist client; do not try to teach client new skills or routines
Level 2: Postural Actions	The client initiates gross body movements, and may maintain bizarre postures. The client may be able to assist in his or her care, but may become distressed or resistive. He or she requires 24-hour supervision.	Structure environment so client can imitate habitual one step gross motor actions like folding towels; do not try to teach client new skills or routines
Level 3: Manual Actions	The client responds to tactile cues, and uses hands to manipulate objects. He or she may engage in repetitive or seemingly pointless actions. The client needs cues to stay on-task, and requires 24-hour supervision.	Long term repetitive training may enable the person to perform simple, routine tasks.

continued

Allen Cognitive Disability Level	Learning Characteristics & Cuing Needed	Intervention Approach
Level 4: Goal-Directed Actions	The person engages in purposeful activity to achieve a short-term goal, in structured environments. He or she can complete routine tasks such as dressing, but requires assistance to solve problems or deal with unexpected situations.	Repetitive practice with living skills specific to person's discharge situation. Simulate actual discharge situation as much as possible as these clients will have difficulty transferring learning across different situations.
Level 5: Exploratory Actions	The client can problem-solve by trial and error, but has difficulty anticipating the results of actions. The client can learn new activities, but needs assistance with activities requiring him or her to plan ahead.	Demonstrate relevant rehabilitation principles and practice; have client apply principles across a variety of functional tasks. E.g., demonstrate transfer techniques and practice applying techniques to different types of transfers (toilet, tub, car, etc.).
Level 6: Planned Actions	The client can anticipate the effects of future actions, and can think abstractly. This makes it possible for him or her to problem-solve and plan future actions in advance. He or she can follow verbal or written instructions without a demonstration.	Client education re: relevant rehabilitation principles; client will be able to practice on own. E.g., education re: principle of using long-handled reacher.

Derived from: Allen, C. K. (1998). Cognitive disability frame of reference. In M. E. Neistadt & E. B. Crepeau (Eds.), *Willard & Spackman's occupational therapy,* 9th ed. (pp. 555–557). Philadelphia: Lippincott, p. 556, with permission. Additional information from Allen, C. K. (1992).

STEP 11   Note type and amount of cuing client needs for activity performance.

The type and amount of cuing clients need is related to their brains' information processing capacities. The information processing capacity of our brains underlies our ability to learn. If the brain cannot process new information—interpret and relate external sensory impressions with internally stored concepts—learning is not possible. All intervention requires client learning. That is, all intervention requires permanent changes in clients' behavior or behavior potential—changes that result from the experience of intervention. The brain must be able to process the experience of intervention if learning is to occur.

Clients who are unable to engage in activity without constant hand-over-hand cuing in the absence of sensory, motor, or perceptual problems that would explain that behavior are demonstrating significant confusion and problems with information processing in the brain. Clients who are having this much trouble processing information will have difficulty learning new, adaptive behaviors. Table 2-21 suggests intervention approaches for the different levels of information processing delineated by Allen's Cognitive Disability Model.

STEP 12   Synthesize and summarize the data; make discharge projections—project and record rehabilitation objectives and interventions planned to reach discharge projections.

SYNTHESIZE AND SUMMARIZE DATA

When you finish your evaluation, you need to synthesize and summarize the data you have gathered into the following: (a) a brief narrative about the client (age, marital status, diagnosis or referring problem, living situation, strengths, and priorities—see Box 2-6 for an example); (b) a problem list that reflects the areas you could work on in occupational therapy; (c) discharge projections (functional level, services, and living situation anticipated after discharge from occupational therapy); and (d) rehabilitation objectives and an intervention plan that will help the client reach the levels of function projected for discharge.

TABLE 2-22 | PROBLEM LIST GUIDE

1) Report ADL Status (levels of assistance required for different ADL tasks—see Box 2.6 for a sample).

2) Write "ADL status due to the following deficits;" and list the deficits that apply from the list below.

Sensation	Motor	Perception	Cognition	Psychosocial
Tactile (specify body parts and degree of impairment, e.g., client reports numbness in toes, both hands)	PROM (specify joints and degrees of limitation or proportion of joint motion absent, eg, R shoulder flexion limited to 1/2 range, PROM)	Motor planning	Attention	Coping skills
Vision (specify visual skills impaired, note whether or not client needs glasses)	AROM for muscle groups with atypical tone (specify joints and degrees of limitation or proportion of joint motion absent, eg, R shoulder flexion limited to 1/2 range, AROM)	Spatial relations	Orientation	Time Management
				continued

TABLE 2-22 | PROBLEM LIST GUIDE (CONTINUED)

1) Report ADL Status (levels of assistance required for different ADL tasks—see Box 2.6 for a sample).

2) Write "ADL status due to the following deficits:" and list the deficits that apply from the list below.

Sensation	Motor	Perception	Cognition	Psychosocial
Hearing (note whether client has difficulty hearing regular conversations, whether or not client needs hearing aid)	Strength, for muscle groups with normal tone (specify by muscle groups and grade, e.g., shoulder flexors limited to 3/5)	Visual discrimination	Sequencing	Self-control
	Endurance (activity tolerance limited to ____ minutes)	Figure-ground	Organization	
	Fine motor coordination		Initiation	
	Gross motor coordination		Memory	
	Postural control (sitting and standing balance, static and dynamic)		Problem-solving	
	Muscle tone; atypical movement patterns		Learning	

Note. ADL = Activities of Daily Living; PROM = passive range of motion; AROM = active range of motion; R = right; See Appendix D for definitions of component skill terms.

The primary focus of occupational therapy is occupation, that is, the day-to-day activities people engage in to fulfill their roles and stay connected to other people. Therefore, your problem list should focus on functional activity deficits and link component skill problems to functional deficits. Table 2-22 suggests one way to do this for narrative notes. The occupational therapy evaluation form at the end of this chapter (Figure 2-29) is an example of a facility's form for summarizing and synthesizing evaluation data.

DISCHARGE PROJECTIONS

In making discharge projections for any given client, you should consider the factors in Figure 2-28.

REHABILITATION OBJECTIVES

Rehabilitation objectives should focus on functional outcomes of value to the client; that is, rehabilitation objectives should focus on

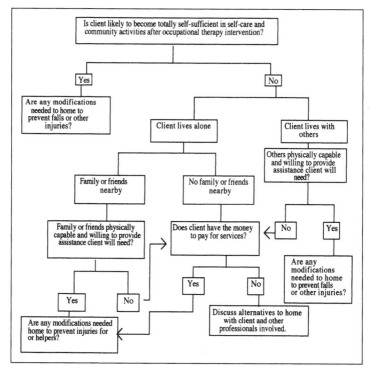

FIGURE 2-28 Discharge Planning Decision Tree

BOX 2-7.	GUIDE TO BEHAVIORAL REHABILITATION OBJECTIVES

All behavioral objectives should have the following elements:

Behavior:	An expected outcome that can be seen or heard (e.g., dressing or speaking)
Criteria:	Expected level of performance (e.g., with minimum assistance or independently)
Conditions:	How the client will perform the behavior (e.g., seated or standing, using adaptive equipment)
Time Frame:	Length of time it will take the client to achieve the target behavior
Example:	Within 1 week, client will:

1) complete LE dressing I-ly using a long-handled reacher while seated.

2) transfering onto toilet I-ly using walker, raising toilet seat, and grab bars.

Behavior:	1) LE dressing; 2) Transfer onto toilet
Criteria:	1 and 2) Independently
Conditions:	1) Using a long-handled reacher while seated
	2) Using walker, raised toilet seat, and grab bars
Time Frame:	1 and 2) Within 1 week

Derived from: Neistadt, M. E. & Crepeau, E. B. (1998). Introduction to occupational therapy. In M. E. Neistadt & E. B. Crepeau (Eds.), *Willard & Spackman's occupational therapy,* 9th ed. (pp. 5–12). Philadelphia: Lippincott, p. 9, with permission.

Note. LE = lower extremity; I = independent.

client behaviors expected as a result of intervention. Behavioral objectives need to be measurable, realistic (appropriate to the client's discharge situation), and attainable within the intervention time allotted, given the client's skill level and anticipated course of recovery. Box 2-7 provides some guidelines for writing behavioral rehabilitation objectives.

INTERVENTIONS

Planned interventions should be clearly linked to the written behavioral objectives; if component skill training is planned, you need to specifically tie it to functional outcomes. For example, "Cognitive retraining to improve client's ability to plan and prepare meals." Intervention also has to be realistic for the client's learning capacity and the number of intervention sessions allotted by the third-party payer.

Figure 2-29 is an example of an occupational therapy evaluation form. A form like this could be used to (a) summarize occupational

FIGURE 2-29 Cedars-Sinai Occupational Therapy Evaluation Profile. Reprinted with permission of Cedars-Sinai Medical Center.

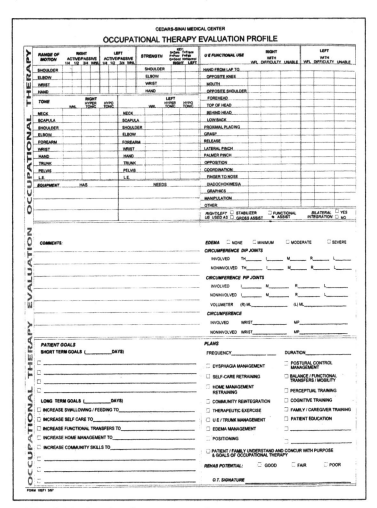

FIGURE 2-29—(continued)

therapy evaluation data, (b) document discharge projections, (c) document clients' rehabilitation objectives, and (d) document an occupational therapy intervention plan. This type of form could also serve as a reminder about the areas to consider in an occupational therapy evaluation.

3
SUGGESTED EVALUATION SEQUENCES FOR DIFFERENT TIME LIMITS

For a variety of reasons, you will not always have time to perform complete occupational therapy (OT) evaluations. Sometimes you may have only 20–30 minutes; in this case, you will need to perform a screening—a brief evaluation to identify a client's need for additional OT evaluation and intervention. This chapter suggests some evaluation sequences for different lengths of time: 20–30 minutes; 30–40 minutes; and 40–60 minutes. Also included in this chapter are suggestions about how to divide an evaluation up throughout several intervention sessions.

In time-pressured evaluation situations, you need to be especially aware of your implicit frame of reference for practice and all of the types of clinical reasoning available to you. The pressures of the moment may encourage you to focus only on completing those procedures necessary to fill out whatever form your facility uses. That is, under time pressure, you may let the form drive your evaluation process and focus primarily on procedural reasoning to identify client's diagnostically related problems. Client's priorities and concerns often get lost in this type of evaluation.

The evaluation process can only yield meaningful information if you approach it with a clear sense of your frame of reference and a firm commitment to meet the person you are evaluating. Your primary objective, no matter how short your evaluation time may be, should be to establish rapport with your client and gain some understanding of what the client wants from the intervention process. This means your interactive reasoning skills need to be particularly sharp for screenings or abbreviated evaluations.

Your narrative reasoning skills must also be sharp for shorter evaluation sessions. You will need to get a preliminary sense of who the client is from only a few questions. Observing and asking about some of the client's personal objects in the evaluation environment may help you build this picture also. For example, just commenting, "What lovely pictures" as you notice photographs on the client's bureau or mantlepiece, might elicit a brief family history that illuminates the client's family roles. If you see a knitted afghan in the client's room, asking, "Did you make this?" could elicit information about the client's leisure interests. A simple question such as, "What kind of work do [or did] you do?" can elicit a vocational history.

In short, no matter how brief your evaluation session, you must think of it as a conversation with the client and include as much actual conversation in the process as possible. Thinking of the evaluation this way will help you to shift back and forth in the session between your procedural, pragmatic, conditional, ethical, narrative, and interactive reasoning. Shifting between all types of clinical reasoning within any evaluation session will help you to (a) identify the problems that are of primary concern to the client and (b) project intervention outcomes that are consistent with the client's usual routines and social supports.

20- TO 30-MINUTE SCREENINGS

Table 3-1 suggests five different ways to proceed with a 20- to 30-minute screening. These suggested options are not the only ways to proceed but will give you some ideas about how to make the most of a short evaluation session with a client. All options incorporate intervention into the screening session; this is important for those third-party payers who will only reimburse for occupational therapy sessions that include intervention. You can follow-up any of these options with additional evaluations interspersed throughout intervention sessions (see pp. 110–113 for suggestions about how to do this).

20- to 30-Minute Screening: Option 1

Box 3-1 provides more detail about Option 1. This option is only feasible if the client or a caregiver can respond to interview questions.

The ADL portion of this screening includes questions to elicit client's ADL priorities. As clients or their caregivers describe clients' difficulties with day-to-day activities in response to other questions, you need to be listening for exactly how clients are having problems with tasks. You will usually need to ask follow-up questions to elicit this information. You might also ask clients to perform some ADL tasks. Tables 3-2 and 3-3 provide some suggestions for follow-up ac-

TABLE 3-1 | OPTIONS FOR 20- TO 30-MINUTE SCREENING

Screening Option	Requires Verbal Communication From Client	Covers BADL	Covers IADL	Includes Intervention
1 ▪ BADL and IADL/client priorities interview ▪ Motor screen ▪ Sensory screen ▪ Cognitive interview	Yes	Yes	Yes	Yes, recommendations for adaptive equipment during ADL interview
2 Mobility evaluation with a physical therapist (have client roll in bed, get out of bed into a chair, ambulate if appropriate, try a toilet transfer if appropriate)	No	Yes	No	Yes, mobility training
3 Observation of shower or other ADL with assistance of an aide	No	Yes	No	Yes, consultation
4 Observation of client at mealtime	No	Yes	No	Yes, consultation
5 Observation of cleaning sink and mirror	No	No	Yes	Yes, consultation and IADL training

BADL = Basic Activities of Daily Living; IADL = Instrumental Activities of Daily Living; ADL = Activities of Daily Living.

BOX 3-1	20- TO 30-MINUTE SCREENING: OPTION 1

Basic and Instrumental Activities of Daily Living/Client Priorities

(Interview client; if client is unable to respond to an interview, talk to primary caregiver.)

- How has **[diagnosis or problem]** affected your day-to-day activities? What sorts of things do you need help with now because of your **[diagnosis or problem]**?
- Do you think **[particular piece of]** adaptive equipment might be helpful to you? Do you already have this equipment?
- Do you think **[a particular]** task method might be helpful to you?
- Which of your day-to-day activities are most important to you?
- Which activities would you most want to do for yourself? Which ones would you feel comfortable delegating to someone else?
- Any problems with sitting, standing, or walking? (Functional mobility)
- How much help do you need for transfers? **[Ask for demonstration]**

Sensory—See Tables 2-13, 2-14, and 2-15 for screening of vision, hearing, and somatic sensation.

Motor See p. 157 for additional detail.

- Hands over head, behind neck and behind back (Active Range of Motion [AROM])
- If AROM limited, Passive Range of Motion (PROM) for limited joints
- Manual Muscle Testing (MMT) of muscle groups
- Rapid motion of each fingertip to thumb (coordination)
- Rapid supination and pronation with arms stretched out in front (coordination)
- Touch therapist's index finger, first with one hand, then the other (motor control)

Cognition (Interview)

- Are you experiencing any problems concentrating or remembering things since your **[diagnosis or problem]**?

tions, observations, and questions you might use for selected BADL and IADL complaints. During your ADL interview, you can also make suggestions about pieces of adaptive equipment (e.g., tub seats and long-handled reachers) or modified task approaches (e.g., sitting down to iron) that might be helpful. By suggesting adaptive equipment and modified task approaches, you are offering consultation and introducing possible intervention strategies. Therefore, Option 1 is a combination of evaluation and intervention.

TABLE 3-2 WAYS TO FOLLOW UP ON CLIENTS' BASIC ACTIVITIES OF DAILY LIVING (BADL) COMPLAINTS DURING AN INTERVIEW

BADL Complaint	Therapist Follow-up Action	Therapist Observations (Possible Component Skill Deficits Indicated)	Therapist Follow-up Questions (Component Skill Addressed)
Trouble with buttoning	If garment with buttons is available, ask client, "Can you try to button this for me?"	▪ Does client use visual guidance for activity? (Somatic sensation or motor planning) ▪ Does client have a tremor during activity? (Muscle weakness or a neurologic tremor) ▪ Are clients' movements awkward? (Motor planning or motor control) ▪ Does client have difficulty initiating the activity? (Cognition) ▪ Does client seem anxious or depressed during activity? (Psychosocial skills)	▪ Is it hard to feel the button? (Sensation) ▪ Are you having trouble seeing the buttons? (Vision/Perception) ▪ Do your fingers feel weak? (Strength) ▪ Do your fingers or arms feel shaky or clumsy? (Motor control/coordination) ▪ Do you have trouble getting started with activities (Initiation) or getting all the steps of the task in the right order? (Sequencing) ▪ Do you feel anxious, tense, or that you just don't want to do this activity? (Psychosocial skills)
Trouble with shirts	If sweater, lab coat, or robe is readily available, ask client,	▪ Does client have difficulty orienting garment? (Spatial perception)	▪ Is it hard to feel the shirt? (Sensation)

continued

TABLE 3-2	WAYS TO FOLLOW UP ON CLIENTS' BASIC ACTIVITIES OF DAILY LIVING (BADL) COMPLAINTS DURING AN INTERVIEW (CONTINUED)

BADL Complaint	Therapist Follow-up Action	Therapist Observations (Possible Component Skill Deficits Indicated)	Therapist Follow-up Questions (Component Skill Addressed)
	"Can you try putting this on for me?" If client able to stand, ask client to do this standing.	■ Does client have difficulty reaching around back or overhead? (Shoulder weakness or limited Passive Range of Motion [PROM]) ■ Does client tend to lose balance during activity? (Balance, muscle weakness in trunk and legs) ■ Also observations under "Trouble with buttoning"	■ Are you having trouble seeing the shirt or figuring out how to get your arms in the sleeves? (Vision/Perception) ■ Also strength, motor control/coordination, initiation and sequencing, and psychosocial questions under "Trouble with buttoning"
Trouble with shoes and socks	Help client take off one shoe and sock and ask, "Can you show me how you try to do this?"	■ Does client have difficulty orienting shoes and socks? (Spatial perception) ■ Does client tend to lose balance during activity? (Balance, muscle weakness in trunk and legs) ■ Does the client have trouble reaching feet? (Limited PROM in hips, lower back) ■ Also observations under "Trouble with buttoning"	■ Is it hard to feel the shoes or socks? (Sensation) ■ Are you having trouble seeing the shoes or socks or figuring out how to get your feet into them? (Vision/Perception) ■ Also strength, motor control/coordination, initiation and sequencing, and psychosocial questions under "Trouble with buttoning"

Note. For additional detail about observations you can make during functional tasks, see Árnadóttir, G. (1990). *The brain and behavior: Assessing cortical dysfunction through tasks of daily living.* St. Louis: The C.V. Mosby Co.

TABLE 3-3 WAYS TO FOLLOW UP ON CLIENTS' INSTRUMENTAL ACTIVITIES OF DAILY LIVING (IADL) COMPLAINTS DURING AN INTERVIEW

IADL Complaint	Therapist Follow-up Action	Therapist Observations (Possible Component Skill Deficits Indicated)	Therapist Follow-up Questions (Component Skill Addressed)
Spilling things	Ask client to try pouring water from one glass to another.	▪ Does client use visual guidance for activity? (Somatic sensation or motor planning) ▪ Does client have difficulty orienting task objects? (Spatial perception) ▪ Does client have a tremor during activity? (Muscle weakness or a neurologic tremor) ▪ Are clients' movements awkward? (Motor planning or motor control) ▪ Does client have difficulty initiating or sequencing the activity? (Cognition) ▪ Does client seem anxious or depressed during activity? (Psychosocial skills)	▪ Is it hard to feel the glasses? (Sensation) ▪ Are you having trouble seeing the glasses or knowing how far apart they are? (Vision/Perception) ▪ Do your arms or fingers feel weak? (Strength) ▪ Do your fingers or arms feel shaky or clumsy? (Motor control/coordination) ▪ Do you have trouble getting started with this activity? (Initiation) getting all the steps of the task in the right order? (Sequencing) ▪ Do you feel anxious, tense, or that you just don't want to do this activity? (Psychosocial skills)
Trouble getting things out of cupboards and closets	Ask client to reach for something on the top shelf of a closet and open the lowest drawer of a bureau.	▪ Does client have difficulty reaching overhead? (Shoulder weakness or limited Passive Range of Motion [PROM])	▪ Is it hard to feel the closet door, drawer, or things you're reaching for? (Sensation) *continued*

TABLE 3-3	WAYS TO FOLLOW-UP ON CLIENTS' INSTRUMENTAL ACTIVITIES OF DAILY LIVING (IADL) COMPLAINTS DURING AN INTERVIEW (CONTINUED)

IADL Complaint	Therapist Follow-up Action	Therapist Observations (Possible Component Skill Deficits Indicated)	Therapist Follow-up Questions (Component Skill Addressed)
		■ Does the client have trouble reaching down to bottom drawer? (Limited PROM in hips, lower back) ■ Does client tend to lose balance during activity? (Balance, muscle weakness in trunk and legs) ■ Also observations under "Spilling things"	■ Are you having trouble seeing the items inside the closet or drawer? (Vision/Perception) ■ Also strength, motor control/ coordination, initiation and sequencing, and psychosocial questions under "Spilling things"
Trouble with using telephone	Ask client to dial his or her own number.	■ Does client use visual guidance for activity? (Somatic sensation or motor planning) ■ Does client have a tremor during activity? (Muscle weakness or a neurologic tremor) ■ Are clients' movements awkward? (Motor planning or motor control) ■ Does client have difficulty initiating or sequencing the activity? (Cognition) ■ Does client seem anxious or depressed during activity? (Psychosocial skills)	■ Is it hard to feel the telephone receiver or buttons? (Sensation) ■ Are you having trouble seeing the telephone receiver, buttons, or numbers? (Vision/Perception) ■ Are you having trouble remembering the number you're dialing? (Cognition) ■ Also strength, motor control/ coordination, initiation and sequencing, and psychosocial questions under "Spilling things"

Note. For additional detail about observations you can make during functional tasks, see Árnadóttir, G. (1990). *The brain and behavior: Assessing cortical dysfunction through tasks of daily living.* St. Louis: The C.V. Mosby Co.

20- to 30-Minute Screening: Option 2

For Option 2, you will be working with a physical therapist to get a client out of bed and into a chair. This type of evaluation might be most appropriate in an acute care setting where clients might have limited ability to move owing to illness or postsurgical pain. In this joint evaluation session, you and the physical therapist will both be observing the client's motor component skills, but you will also be contributing observations about the client's visual, auditory, and perceptual/cognitive skills. The physical therapist will be focused on standing and ambulation; you will be more focused on transfers and the client's cognitive ability to use mobility devices, such as walkers.

This option is activity-based, not interview-based, and therefore is feasible if the client has communication difficulties. If the client does have communication difficulties, you will have to get information about the client's priorities from family members, friends, or caregivers. However, if the client is able to communicate, you could ask about the client's activity priorities before you begin helping the client to move. Box 3-2 provides an introduction that incorporates this question into the session.

The observations you make in Option 2 form the basis for both your evaluation and a consultation with other caregivers about how to best help this particular client to move. Thus, Option 2 is a combination of evaluation and intervention.

Table 3-4 provides a summary of selected component skill observations you might make during this functional mobility session; this table does not detail all possible observations because it is meant only to trigger your knowledge of activity analysis. Chapter 2 provides more detail about looking for component skill deficits during clients' func-

BOX 3-2	INTRODUCTION FOR BED MOBILITY SCREENING

Hello, Mr. or Ms. **[name]**. I am **[name]** from occupational therapy and this is [*name*] from physical therapy. We are here to help you get up out of bed. We understand this will not be easy for you but we are here to help you. Getting up out of bed is important to help you start moving around more. If client is unable to communicate, continue with explanation, instructions about how you would like the client to begin moving.

If client is alert and can communicate, before beginning to move him or her, you could ask, "When you were able to move better, which of your day-to-day activities were really important to you?" **[client response]**. Well, this is the first step to getting back to **[activity identified by client]**. Continue with explanation, including instructions about how you would like the client to begin moving.

CHAPTER 3

TABLE 3-4 SUMMARY OF SELECTED COMPONENT SKILL OBSERVATIONS FOR FUNCTIONAL MOBILITY

Functional Mobility Activities	Sensory Skills (Related Behavior)	Perceptual Skills (Related Behavior)	Cognitive Skills (Related Behavior)	Motor Skills (Related Behavior)	Psychosocial Skills (Related Behavior)
Bed mobility and transfers	■ Vision (able to scan across environment, see bedrail, arm of chair) ■ Auditory (asking for repetition of or louder verbal cues) ■ Somatic (unable to grasp bedrail or arm of chair)	■ Unilateral neglect (moves as if left or right side of body did not exist) ■ Motor planning (awkward movements) ■ Spatial skills (misses bedrail or armchair when reaching for them)	■ Attention (distracted by noise) ■ Concentration (unable to complete task without cuing; needs one step cues) ■ Sequencing (does steps of task out of order) ■ Initiation (unable to begin task without cuing) ■ Judgment (does not put self at risk for falling)	■ Balance (does not lose) ■ Strength and Flexibility (able to roll, push up to sitting on side of bed, support weight on legs) ■ Coordination (smooth movements of arms and legs)	■ Affect (shows frustration, humor, etc. appropriately) ■ Interpersonal skills (interacts appropriately with therapists)

Note. For additional detail about observations you can make during functional tasks, see Árnadóttir, G. (1990). *The brain and behavior: Assessing cortical dysfunction through tasks of daily living.* St. Louis: The C.V. Mosby Co.

tional activity performances and may further trigger recall of your knowledge base.

20- to 30-Minute Screening: Option 3

For Option 3, you will be observing the client during part of an ADL session with a home health or nursing aide. Before doing this, you need to be very clear with both the client and the aide that you are observing to try to see what types of problems the client is having with ADL. The aide should not feel that you are there to critique his or her performance. You also need to clarify at the beginning of your observation session that you will be sharing your observations with both the client and aide at the next session. You want to establish a collaborative working relationship with both the client and the aide—open sharing of information is essential to that relationship. Providing practical assistance where needed during the session, for example, helping with a transfer or handing the aide a shampoo bottle that is out of reach, will also help establish a collaborative relationship with the client and aide.

This option is activity-based, not interview-based, and so is feasible if the client has communication difficulties. If the client does have communication difficulties, you will have to get information about the client's priorities from family members, friends, or caregivers. However, if the client is able to communicate and is not distracted by talking during the ADL session, you could talk to the client during this session asking him or her about which day-to-day activities are most important to do independently and for which ones he or she would like to get help.

The observations you make in Option 3 form the basis for both your evaluation and a consultation with the aide about how to best work with this particular client. That is, your observations will allow you to (a) explain to the aide how the client's particular component skill difficulties contribute to the client's behaviors during ADL, (b) suggest particular types of cuing that might be especially helpful for this client, and (c) suggest ways to arrange the activity objects and environment that will facilitate client performance. Therefore, Option 3 is a combination of evaluation and intervention.

Table 3-5 provides a summary of selected component skill observations you might make during shower or dressing activities; this table does not cover all possible observations because it is meant only to trigger your knowledge of activity analysis. Chapter 2 provides more detail about looking for component skill deficits during clients' functional activity performances and may further trigger recall of your knowledge base.

CHAPTER 3

TABLE 3-5	SUMMARY OF SELECTED COMPONENT SKILL OBSERVATIONS FOR BASIC ACTIVITIES OF DAILY LIVING (BADL) ACTIVITIES

BADL Activity	Sensory Skills (Related Behavior)	Perceptual Skills (Related Behavior)	Cognitive Skills (Related Behavior)	Motor Skills (Related Behavior)	Psychosocial Skills (Related Behavior)
Dressing	▪ Vision (squinting, moving objects close or far from eyes to focus on them; scanning) ▪ Auditory (asking for repetition of or louder verbal cues) ▪ Somatic (dropping objects)	▪ Unilateral neglect (only dresses left or right side of body) ▪ Motor planning (awkward movements, misplacement of garments on body) ▪ Spatial skills (difficulty putting arms and legs in correct holes in garments, etc.)	▪ Attention (distracted by noise) ▪ Concentration (unable to complete task without cuing; needs one step cues) ▪ Sequencing (does steps of task out of order) ▪ Initiation (unable to begin task without cuing) ▪ Judgment (chooses clothes appropriate to weather)	▪ Balance (does not lose) ▪ Strength and flexibility (able to reach, hold objects) ▪ Coordination (able to manipulate objects)	▪ Affect (shows frustration, humor, etc., appropriately) ▪ Interpersonal skills (interacts appropriately with caregivers)
Showering	▪ Vision (squinting, moving objects close or far from eyes to focus on them; scanning) ▪ Auditory (asking for repetition of or louder verbal cues)	▪ Unilateral neglect (only washes left or right side of body) ▪ Motor planning (awkward movements, misuse of task objects) ▪ Spatial skills (difficulty	▪ Attention (distracted by noise) ▪ Concentration (unable to complete task without cueing) ▪ Sequencing (does steps of task out of order)	▪ Balance (does not lose) ▪ Strength and flexibility (able to reach, hold objects) ▪ Coordination (able to manipulate objects)	▪ Affect (shows frustration, humor, etc., appropriately) ▪ Interpersonal skills (interacts appropriately with caregivers)

	▪ Somatic (dropping objects)	putting soap and wash-cloth together, etc.)	▪ Initiation (unable to begin task without cuing) ▪ Judgment (does not put self at risk for falling)		▪ Affect (shows frustration, humor, etc., appropriately) ▪ Interpersonal skills (interacts appropriately with caregivers)
Mealtime	▪ Vision (squinting, moving objects close or far from eyes to focus on them; scanning) ▪ Auditory (asking for repetition of or louder verbal cues) ▪ Somatic (dropping objects)	▪ Unilateral neglect (only eats food on left or right side of plate) ▪ Motor planning (awkward movements, misuse of utensils) ▪ Spatial skills (spills sugar, difficulty putting glass down in a clear space on table, etc.)	▪ Attention (distracted by noise) ▪ Concentration (unable to complete task without cuing) ▪ Sequencing (does steps of task out of order) ▪ Initiation (unable to begin task without cuing) ▪ Judgment (does not put too much food in mouth or eat too quickly)	▪ Balance (does not lose) ▪ Strength and flexibility (able to reach, hold objects) ▪ Coordination (able to manipulate objects)	

Note. For additional detail about observations you can make during functional tasks, see Árnadóttir, G. (1990). *The brain and behavior: Assessing cortical dysfunction through tasks of daily living.* St. Louis: The C.V. Mosby Co.

20- to 30-Minute Screening: Option 4

For Option 4, you will be observing the client during a mealtime. In some settings, you might complete this observation in conjunction with a speech and language pathologist who would be making observations relative to the client's chewing and swallowing abilities. For this observation, you need to ask the client if it is all right for you to visit with him or her during lunch. Mealtime is often a social event and no one wants to feel like they're being watched while they're eating. So you need to present this observation as a visit, indicating that while you are visiting, you will be noting what kind of help the client needs with eating and providing any help that is needed.

Option 4 is activity-based, not interview-based, and so is feasible if the client has communication difficulties. If the client does have communication difficulties, you will have to get information about the client's priorities from family members, friends, or caregivers. However, if the client is able to communicate and not distracted by conversation during the meal, you ask about the client's vocational history, typical routines, and activity priorities while he or she is eating.

The observations you make in Option 4 form the basis for both your evaluation and your recommendations about the kinds of assistance and set-up a client might need with meals. Therefore, Option 4 is a combination of evaluation and intervention.

Table 3-5 provides a summary of selected component skill observations you might make during this cleaning activity; this table does not cover all possible observations because it is meant only to trigger your knowledge of activity analysis. Chapter 2 provides more detail about looking for component skill deficits during clients' functional activity performances and may further trigger recall of your own knowledge base.

20- to 30-Minute Screening: Option 5

For Option 5, you will be observing the client performing the IADL task of cleaning a sink and mirror. For this observation, you need to tell the client, "I am here to figure out what difficulties your diagnostically related problems are creating for you in day-to-day activities. To do this, I need to see you actually try a common daily activity. I'd like you to try cleaning the sink and the mirror over the sink. I will help you if you need help."

Option 5 would be most appropriate for clients who are (a) ambulatory, (b) not showing significant BADL problems according to caregivers or client records, (c) typically engaged in housekeeping responsibilities, and (d) likely to have a short course of therapy. Option 5 is activity-based, not interview-based, and therefore is feasible if the client has communication difficulties. If the client does have communication difficulties, you will have to get information about the client's priorities from family members, friends, or caregivers. However, if the client is able to communicate and not distracted by conversation, you could ask about the client's vocational history, typical routines, and activity priorities while he or she is cleaning the sink and mirror.

The observations you make in Option 5 form the basis for both your evaluation and your recommendations about the kinds of assistance and set-up a client might need with homemaking tasks. Therefore, Option 5 is a combination of evaluation and intervention.

Table 3-6 provides a summary of selected component skill observations you might make during this cleaning activity; this table does not cover all possible observations because it is meant only to trigger your knowledge of activity analysis. Chapter 2 provides more detail about looking for component skill deficits during clients' functional activity performances and may further trigger recall of your own knowledge base.

30- TO 40-MINUTE EVALUATIONS

If you have 30–40 minutes for you initial evaluation, you may be able to have a client do more BADL or IADL activities than in a 20- to 30-minute session. However, you will still not have enough time to complete a full morning BADL routine or full kitchen evaluation for most clients. Clients with serious motor problems, confusion, or slowed information processing will need longer periods of time to carry out activities. Additionally, if you are evaluating clients in environments that are unfamiliar to them, activities will take longer than usual. Think about how inefficient you are when trying to make a cup of coffee in someone else's kitchen. In an unfamiliar environment, we need extra time just to figure out where things are; in some cases, we may need to come up with very different methods of doing our usual tasks (e.g., taking a bed bath instead of a shower). Rushing clients to meet your time deadlines will give you neither an accurate picture of how much time the client needs nor what the client can do for him or herself when given enough time.

Table 3-7 suggests two different ways to proceed with a 30- to 40-minute evaluation. These suggested options are not the only ways to proceed but will give you some ideas about how to make the most of

| TABLE 3-6 | SUMMARY OF SELECTED COMPONENT SKILL OBSERVATIONS FOR A CLEANING ACTIVITY |

IADL Activity	Sensory Skills (Related Behavior)	Perceptual Skills (Related Behavior)	Cognitive Skills (Related Behavior)	Motor Skills (Related Behavior)	Psychosocial Skills (Related Behavior)
Cleaning a sink and mirror	▪ Vision (squinting, moving close or far from sink or mirror to see them clearly, scans only part of sink and mirror) ▪ Auditory (asking for repetition of or louder verbal cues) ▪ Somatic (dropping objects)	▪ Unilateral neglect (only cleans left or right side of sink and mirror) ▪ Motor planning (awkward movements) ▪ Spatial skills (misses sink or mirror when squirting cleaning solution, etc.)	▪ Attention (distracted by noise) ▪ Concentration (unable to complete task without cuing; needs one-step cues) ▪ Sequencing (does steps of task out of order) ▪ Initiation (unable to begin task without cuing) ▪ Judgment (recognizes when sink and mirror are clean, does not put self at risk of falling)	▪ Balance (does not lose) ▪ Strength and flexibility (able to reach top of mirror and under sink, able to hold cleaning solution and cloth) ▪ Coordination (able to manipulate cleaning solution and cloth)	▪ Affect (shows frustration, humor, etc. appropriately) ▪ Interpersonal skills (interacts appropriately with therapist)

Note. For additional detail about observations you can make during functional tasks, see Árnadóttir, G. (1990). *The brain and behavior: Assessing cortical dysfunction through tasks of daily living.* St. Louis: The C.V. Mosby Co.
IADL = Instrumental Activities of Daily Living.

TABLE 3-7	OPTIONS FOR 30- TO 40-MINUTE EVALUATIONS

Evaluation Option	Requires Verbal Communication From Client	Covers BADL	Covers IADL	Includes Intervention
1 ■ Part of morning BADL routine (e.g., dressing or grooming) ■ Client priorities interview (see Appendix A) ■ Sensory screen ■ Motor screen ■ Cognitive interview (see Box 3-1) or Mini-Mental State (MMS) (see Appendix D for information)	No, for BADL Yes, for rest of evaluation	Yes	No	Yes, BADL training
2 ■ Have client make cup of tea or coffee in kitchen ■ Client priorities interview (see Appendix A) ■ Sensory screen ■ Motor screen ■ Cognitive interview (see Box 3.1) or Mini-Mental State (MMS) (see Appendix D for information)	No, for IADL Yes, for rest of evaluation	No	No	Yes, IADL training

BADL = Basic Activities of Daily Living; IADL = Instrumental Activities of Daily Living.

a 30- to 40-minute evaluation session with a client. Both options include a client priorities interview. Taking some time in your evaluation sessions to get this information will help you (a) design intervention that is meaningful to the client and (b) make accurate predictions of client function after intervention. Therefore, the time spent learning about client priorities is well spent and more important than completing a more extensive BADL or IADL routine.

Both options in Table 3-7 also incorporate intervention into the evaluation session via functional skills training; this is important for those third-party payers who will only reimburse for occupational therapy sessions that include intervention. When clients are slow in performing functional tasks, you may not have time for the other interviews and screenings suggested for both options. You can follow-up either of these options with additional screenings or evaluations in-

CHAPTER 3

terspersed throughout intervention sessions (see p. 110–113 for suggestions about how to do this).

Both options in Table 3-7 include both activity-based portions (e.g., BADL or IADL activities) and interview portions (e.g., client priorities and cognitive interviews). The activity-based portions of Options 1 and 2 may not pose problems for clients with communication problems. However, you will have to modify the interview and screening procedures for clients with communication problems. Box 3-3 provides some suggestions for ways to do this. For clients without communication or cognitive problems who have no problem talking while they are doing functional tasks, you could save time by informally interviewing such clients about their priorities and life histories during the activity portion of Options 1 and 2, using the initial interview suggestions in Chapter 2 (see p. 32).

BOX 3-3	MODIFICATIONS OF EVALUATION PROCEDURES FOR ADULT WITH COMMUNICATION PROBLEMS

1) Use gesture and demonstration of instructions. For example:
   - Show client AROM testing sequence by performing the motions yourself.
   - Show client pictures of screening procedures in this or other books

2) Provide client with multiple choice options for pointing responses. For example:
   - Show client pictures of different daily activities and ask client to point to the ones that are most important to him or her.
   - For somatic sensory testing, have client open eyes after the stimuli and point to place you just touched.

3) Keep your explanations short and simple, and augment with gestures if client is having difficulty processing auditory input. For example:
   - "I am going to see how strong you are." Make a muscle with your biceps.
   - "I need to test your feeling." Stroke you arm, turn on the hot water at a sink, touch the water and pull away saying "hot."

4) Phrase questions in yes/no format for clients who are able to use "yes" and "no" accurately. For example:
   - Do you cook at home?
   - Did you feel that? (somatic sensory screening)

5) Check with speech and language pathologist on the intervention team for suggestions to optimize communication with clients with speech and language problems. For example:
   - Does client have a communication book or augmentative communication device?
   - Is client able to use "yes" and "no" accurately and reliably?

30- to 40-Minute Evaluation: Option 1

For Option 1, you will need to negotiate with nursing or home health aides or caregivers to help the client with that portion of the morning BADL routine you do not plan to do with the client. During this negotiation, you need to be clear that you are there to evaluate the client's problems in doing the BADL for him or herself, not simply to help the client complete the morning routine. Alternately, you could plan to give the client maximum assistance with some portions of the BADL routine so the client will finish this routine within 40 minutes. In some situations, you may be able to coordinate your session with a physical therapist so that the physical therapist works with the client right before your session, getting the client out of bed and perhaps even sitting at a sink. Then, you would be free to focus on bathing and dressing with the client.

Table 3-5 provides a summary of selected component skill observations you might make during a shower or dressing activities; this table does not cover all possible observations because it is meant only to trigger your knowledge of activity analysis. Chapter 2 provides more detail about looking for component skill deficits during clients' functional activity performances and may further trigger recall of your knowledge base.

30- to 40-Minute Evaluation: Option 2

For Option 2, you will need access to a kitchen. That kitchen must be supplied with tea bags, instant coffee, milk, sugar, mugs, and a pot or kettle to boil water. Table 3-8 provides a summary of selected component skill observations you might make during this kitchen activity; this table does not cover all possible observations because it is meant only to trigger your knowledge of activity analysis. Chapter 2 provides more detail about looking for component skill deficits during clients' functional activity performances and may further trigger recall of your knowledge base.

40- TO 60-MINUTE EVALUATIONS

If you have 40–60 minutes for your initial evaluation, you can have a client do more BADL or IADL activities than in a 30- to 40-minute session. However, 60 minutes may still not be enough time for some clients to complete a morning BADL routine or full kitchen evaluation.

CHAPTER 3

TABLE 3-8	SUMMARY OF SELECTED COMPONENT SKILL OBSERVATIONS FOR MEAL PREPARATION

IADL Activity	Sensory Skills (Related Behavior)	Perceptual Skills (Related Behavior)	Cognitive Skills (Related Behavior)	Motor Skills (Related Behavior)	Psychosocial Skills (Related Behavior)
Making a hot instant beverage, a sandwich, or a salad	■ Vision (squinting, moving close or far from objects, stove dials to see them clearly, scans only part of environment) ■ Auditory (asking for repetition of or louder verbal cues) ■ Somatic (dropping objects)	■ Unilateral neglect (misses items on left or right side of shelves) ■ Motor planning (awkward movements) ■ Spatial skills (misses cup when adding milk or sugar, etc.)	■ Attention (distracted by noise) ■ Concentration (unable to complete task without cuing; needs one step cues) ■ Sequencing (does steps of task out of order) ■ Initiation (unable to begin task without cuing) ■ Judgment (turns off stove after water boils, does not put self at risk for burns or falling)	■ Balance (does not lose) ■ Strength and flexibility (able to reach high and low shelves in cupboards and refrigerator, able to hold cups, plates, containers) ■ Coordination (able to open containers, work stove dials, cut vegetables, etc.)	■ Affect (shows frustration, humor, etc. appropriately) ■ Interpersonal skills (interacts appropriately with therapist)

Note. For additional detail about observations you can make during functional tasks, see Árnadóttir, G. (1990). *The brain and behavior: Assessing cortical dysfunction through tasks of daily living.* St. Louis: The C.V. Mosby Co.
IADL = Instrumental Activities of Daily Living.

Table 3-9 suggests two different ways to proceed with a 40- to 60-minute evaluation. These suggested options are not the only ways to proceed, but they will give you some ideas about how to make the most of a 40- to 60-minute evaluation session with a client. Both options include a client priorities interview. Taking some time in your evaluation sessions to get this information will help you (a) design intervention meaningful to the client and (b) make accurate predictions of the client's function after intervention. Therefore, the time spent on learn-

| **TABLE 3-9** | OPTIONS FOR 40- TO 60-MINUTE EVALUATIONS |

Evaluation Option	**Requires Verbal Communication From Client**	**Covers BADL**	**Covers IADL**	**Includes Intervention**
1 ▪ Entire morning BADL routine (bathing, grooming, dressing) ▪ Client priorities interview (see Appendix A) ▪ Sensory screen ▪ Motor screen ▪ Cognitive interview (see Box 3.1) or Mini-Mental State (MMS) (see Appendix D for information)	No, for BADL Yes, for rest of evaluation	Yes	No	Yes, BADL training
2 ▪ Have client make a sandwich and a hot beverage (Rabideau Kitchen Evaluation-Revised—see Appendix B for information) or ▪ Have client prepare fruit or vegetable salad and beverage ▪ Client priorities interview (see Appendix A) ▪ Sensory screen ▪ Motor screen ▪ Cognitive interview (see Box 3-1) or Mini-Mental State (MMS) (see Appendix D for information)	No, for IADL Yes, for rest of evaluation	No	Yes	Yes, IADL training

BADL = Basic Activities of Daily Living; IADL = Instrumental Activities of Daily Living.

CHAPTER 3

ing about client priorities is well spent and more important than completing a more extensive BADL or IADL routine.

Both options also incorporate intervention into the evaluation session via functional skills training; this is important for those third-party payers who will only reimburse for occupational therapy sessions that include intervention. When clients are slow in performing functional tasks, you may not have time for the other interviews and screenings suggested for both options. You can follow-up either of these options with additional screenings or evaluations interspersed throughout intervention sessions (see p. 110–113 for suggestions about how to do this).

Both options in Table 3-9 include both activity-based portions (e.g., BADL or IADL activities) and interview portions (e.g., client priorities and cognitive interviews). The activity portions of Options 1 and 2 may not pose problems for clients with communication problems. However, you will have to modify the interview and screening procedures for clients with communication problems. Box 3-3 provides some suggestions for ways to do this. For clients without communication or cognitive problems who have no problem talking while they are doing functional tasks, you could save time by informally interviewing them about their priorities and life histories during the activity portion of Options 1 and 2, using the initial interview suggestions in Chapter 2 (see p. 32).

Tables 3-5 and 3-8 provide summaries of selected component skill observations you might make during BADL or kitchen activities; these tables do not cover all possible observations because they are meant only to trigger your knowledge of activity analysis. Chapter 2 provides more detail about looking for component skill deficits during clients' functional activity performances and may further trigger recall of your knowledge base.

DOING AN EVALUATION DURING THE COURSE OF SEVERAL INTERVENTION SESSIONS

Most often, your initial meeting with a client will give you only a general idea of the client's problems, that is, sufficient information to suggest an intervention plan to the client. To get further detail about the client's problems, you will need to do additional testing during intervention sessions. The best way to do this is to use a few minutes of intervention sessions for evaluation and the rest for intervention. Box 3-4 lists some BADL and IADL activities that you and the client could possibly complete within 20–25 minutes, leaving 5–10 minutes of a

BOX 3-4	SOME INTERVENTION ACTIVITIES FOR 20 TO 25 MINUTES

Basic Activities of Daily Living (BADL)

- Grooming (washing face at sink, brushing teeth, combing hair)
- Shaving face
- Putting on makeup
- Filing or cutting fingernails
- Dressing—with clothes laid out by therapist
- Getting out of bed and into a chair for breakfast

Instrumental Activities of Daily Living (IADL)

- Making tea, instant coffee, or instant hot chocolate
- Making a bed
- Watering plants
- Dusting furniture in one room
- Mopping a floor
- Folding laundry

Note. These intervention activities can be combined with one or two of the formal evaluations listed in Box 3-6, within a 30-minute session.

BOX 3-5	SOME INTERVENTION ACTIVITIES FOR 40 TO 45 MINUTES

Basic Activities of Daily Living (BADL)

- Showering and dressing (clothes laid out by therapist)
- Shaving face, flossing and brushing teeth, combing hair
- Tweezing eyebrows, putting on makeup
- Polishing nails
- Dressing, including getting clothes from closet and drawers
- Getting out of bed and toileting

Instrumental Activities of Daily Living (IADL)

- Making a small meal (sandwich, salad)
- Changing the sheets on a bed
- Repotting a plant
- Cleaning a bathroom sink and toilet
- Vacuuming rug in one room
- Taking laundry out of a dryer and folding it

Note. These intervention activities can be combined with several of the formal evaluations listed in Box 3-6, within a 60-minute session.

30-minute session for some evaluation. Box 3-5 lists some BADL and IADL activities that you and the client could possibly complete within 40–45 minutes, leaving 15–20 minutes of a 60-minute session for some evaluation. You will be the best judge of (a) which intervention activities might be most meaningful and helpful for any given client and (b) how much time that client will need to complete particular intervention activities.

BOX 3-6	FORMAL EVALUATIONS FOR 5 TO 10 MINUTES

Client Priorities

- Part of Canadian Occupational Performance Measure (e.g, Priorities for Self-care, Productivity, or Leisure, or all three if time permits; Performance and Satisfaction Scoring another day)
- Part of Occupational Self-assessment (e.g, form for "Myself" one day, form for "My Environment" another day)

Sensation

- Somatic sensory testing (see Appendix C)—one or two types of sensation in 5–10 minutes
- Full visual screening (see Table 2-13)

Perception and Cognition (Appendix D)

- Mini-Mental State
- Subtests for LOTCA or LOTCA-G, in order—as many as can be completed in 10 minutes; full evaluation will be complete over several intervention sessions

Motor (Appendix E)

- Manual Muscle Testing (MMT)—as many tests as can be completed in 10 minutes
- Fine motor coordination test (e.g., Purdue Pegboard) subtests over successive days
- Formal balance test (e.g., Tinetti Balance and Gait Evaluation) subtests over successive days

Psychosocial

- Allen Cognitive Level Test-90 (ACLS-90)
- Kohlman Evaluation of Living Skills (KELS) subtests, in order, on successive days
- Milwaukee Evaluation of Daily Living Skills (MEDLS) subtests on successive days

Discharge

- Parts of formal interview over successive days

Boxes 3-4 and 3-5 focus on functional activities because nearly all clients will need to practice functional activities to achieve functional goals. Focusing on functional activities will be especially important if you have only a few sessions to work with a client.

Box 3-6 lists segments of evaluations you could complete within 5–10 minutes. The idea is to combine activities from Boxes 3-4 or 3-5 and 3-6. You want to spend at least two thirds of any intervention session on intervention, with no more than one third of the session spent on formal evaluation. You will, of course, be doing informal evaluation throughout any intervention session via observation and activity analysis. Boxes 3-4, 3-5, and 3-6 are not exhaustive because they are only meant to stimulate your thinking about how to manage intervention and formal evaluation time within one session.

CHAPTER 3

A

INTERVIEW ASSESSMENTS OF CLIENT PRIORITIES

ACTIVITY INDEX AND MEANINGFULNESS OF ACTIVITY SCALE

Purpose

The Activity Index (Gregory, 1983) checklist was designed to tap activity interest and participation for older adults. The Meaningfulness of Activity Scale (Gregory, 1983) was designed to tap feelings of enjoyment, autonomy, and competence relative to activities for older adults.

Description

The Activity Index (Gregory, 1983) contains 24 activity items, 2 related to work, 21 related to leisure, and 1 for "Other." For each item, the client places a check in one of four columns: "Don't Do/Not Interested"; "Don't Do/Would Like To"; "Do at Least Once a Week"; "Do at Least Three Times a Week." Checks in the first two columns are valued 0, checks in the third column are valued 1, and those in the fourth column are valued 2. The potential score range is 0 to 52.

The Meaningfulness of Activity Scale (Gregory, 1983) lists the same 24 activity items but asks the client to rank only those activities done one or more times per week. For each of those activities, clients are asked to indicate their enjoyment, autonomy, and competence with

With the exception of ordering information, unless otherwise noted, the information in this appendix has been modified and reprinted with permission from: Henry, A. (1998). The interview process in occupational therapy. In M. E. Neistadt & E. B. Crepeau (Eds.), *Willard & Spackman's occupational therapy* (pp. 155–168). Philadelphia: Lippincott.

Likert-type scales. The potential score range is 78 to 234. (Description not from Henry [1998])

Method

Both are paper-and-pencil self-report measures. A client can complete the checklists on his or her own. However, it is best for you to be present when the client completes the self-report measure, to ensure that the client comprehends what is being asked and is responding appropriately.

Psychometric Properties

Total scores on both measures demonstrated good test–retest reliability with small pilot samples (0.70 and 0.87, respectively). Scores on both measures were also found to positively correlate with a measure of life satisfaction.

Ordering Information

Available in: Gregory, M. D. (1983). Occupational behavior and life satisfaction among retirees. *American Journal of Occupational Therapy, 37,* 548–553.

ADOLESCENT LEISURE INTEREST PROFILE (ALIP)

Purpose

The Adolescent Leisure Interest Profile (ALIP) (Henry, 1996) was designed to tap leisure interests, leisure participation, and feelings about leisure among adolescents.

Description

Henry (1996), adapted the scales developed by Gregory (1983), to develop this measure of leisure interest for adolescents. The checklist contains 86 items about adolescent leisure activities.

Method

The ALIP is a paper-and-pencil self-report measure. A client can complete the checklist on his or her own. However, it is best for you to be present when the client completes the self-report measure, to ensure that the client comprehends what is being asked and is responding appropriately.

Psychometric Properties

Preliminary studies with both normal adolescents and adolescents with disabilities indicate that the ALIP total scores demonstrate good test–retest reliability.

Ordering Information

Currently in press. Contact Alexis Henry via e-mail for more information: alexis.henry@banyan.ummed.edu

ADOLESCENT ROLE ASSESSMENT (ARA)

Purpose

The Adolescent Role Assessment (ARA) (Black, 1976) was designed to provide information about an adolescent's involvement in different occupational roles over time.

Description

The ARA (Black, 1976) is the only occupational therapy interview specifically targeted for adolescents. The 21 questions of the ARA cover six areas: childhood play, socialization within the family, school functioning, socialization with peers, occupational choice, and anticipated adult work. The items are scored with a 3-point scale; (+) indicates appropriate behavior, (0) indicates marginal or borderline behavior, (−) indicates inappropriate behavior.

Method

This assessment is a semi-structured interview.

Psychometric Properties

Black (1982) reported a test–retest reliability coefficient of 0.91 for the rating scale in a pilot study with a small group of adolescents. In addi-

APPENDIX A

tion, the scores on the ARA were found to discriminate between psychiatrically hospitalized adolescents (n = 12) and nonhospitalized adolescents drawn from a high school (n = 28). The ARA appears to yield useful information regarding an adolescent's functioning in occupations.

Ordering Information

Available in: Black, M.M. (1976). Adolescent Role Assessment. *American Journal of Occupational Therapy, 30,* 73–79.

NPI INTEREST CHECKLIST

Purpose

The NPI Interest Checklist (Matsutsuyu, 1969) was designed to indicate a client's level of interest in a range of activities.

Description

The NPI interest checklist contains 80 activity items, which can be grouped in five categories: activities of daily living, manual skills, cultural/educational activities, physical sports, and social/recreational activities. In completing the checklist, the client indicates strong, casual, or no interest in the activity (Rogers, 1988). Kielhofner and Neville (1983) modified the NPI interest checklist to include questions regarding changes in activity preferences over time, and the desire to participate in interests in the future.

Method

The NPI interest checklist is paper-and-pencil self-report measure. A client can complete the checklist on his or her own. However, it is best for you to be present when the client completes the self-report measure, to ensure that the client comprehends what is being asked and is responding appropriately.

Psychometric Properties

Test–retest reliability of the NPI interest checklist was examined by Weinstein (1979). Using a 5-point Likert-type scale, a reliability coefficient of 0.92 was obtained. Two studies have found scores on the interest checklist to discriminate between normal and psychosocially dysfunctional adolescents (Barris, et al., 1986; Ebb, Coster & Duncombe, 1989). Moreover, Henry (1994) found variables derived from the NPI Interest Checklist that reflect an interest in recreational activities to be predictive of functioning for adolescents and young adults with psychosis following hospitalization.

Ordering Information

Available in: Matsutsuyu, J. (1969). The interest checklist. *American Journal of Occupational Therapy, 23,* 323–328.

OCCUPATIONAL SELF-ASSESSMENT (OSA)

Purpose

The OSA (Baron, Kielhofner, Goldhammer, & Wolenski, 1998) was designed to "capture clients' perceptions of their own occupational competence and the impact of their environment on their occupational adaptation" (Baron et al., 1998, p.1). It is used to facilitate collaborative goal setting with clients. The OSA is considered most useful for clients at higher functional levels who have some insight, sufficient cognitive skills to engage in self-reflection and planning, and a desire to work collaboratively with a therapist.

Description

The OSA consists of two occupational self assessment forms—one for self and one for environment. The assessment form for self lists a series of statements related to things people do everyday, e.g., concentrating on tasks, getting along with others, getting done what I need to, doing activities I like. For each occupational functioning statement, clients circle responses that characterize their performance in that area (strength, adequate functioning, or weakness) and the importance of that area to them (extremely important, important, not very important). Then the client goes back and decides on four occupational functioning areas he or she would like to change, and prioritizes those goals. The assessment form for environment lists a series of statements related to living and work environments things, e.g., a place to live and take care of myself, the things I need to be productive, people who encourage and support me. Similar to the first form, clients have to indicate whether these items are problems, how important they are, and what two items they would like to change. Forms are provided for therapists and clients to record client goals and plans of action. Summary forms for clients' demographics, initial assessment and discharge assessment are also provided (Figure A-1).

OSA Data Summary Sheet: Admission to Occupational Therapy Program

Myself	Competence			Values			
	problem	all right	well	not so important	important	extremely important	Priority
Concentrating on my tasks.							
Physically doing what I need to do.							
Taking care of the place where I live.							
Taking care of myself.							
Taking care of others for whom I am responsible.							
Getting where I need to go.							
Managing my finances.							
Managing my basic needs (food, medicine).							
Expressing myself to others.							
Getting along with others.							
Identifying and solving problems.							
Relaxing and enjoying myself.							
Getting done what I need to do.							
Having a satisfying routine.							
Handling my responsibilities.							
Being involved as a student, worker, volunteer, and/or family member.							
Doing activities I like.							
Working towards my goals.							
Making decisions based on what I think is important.							
Accomplishing what I set out to do.							
Effectively using my abilities.							

Date:
Therapist:
Client:

Informed Consent Status:
☐ Informed consent obtained and attached
☐ Informed consent obtained and on client record
☐ Interview collected as part of clinical data and submitted for secondary analysis
Translation used? ☐ No ☐ Yes, used:
☐ Chinese ☐ German
☐ Danish ☐ Icelandic
☐ Dutch ☐ Japanese
☐ Finnish ☐ Portuguese
☐ Flemish-Dutch ☐ Spanish
☐ French ☐ Swedish
Age:
Gender: ☐ M ☐ F
Ethnicity:
☐ Caucasian
☐ African American
☐ Asian/Pacific Islander
☐ American Indian or Alaskan Native
☐ Hispanic
☐ Multiracial
☐ Other _____
☐ Unknown
Diagnosis/ICD9 Code:
Primary:
Secondary:

Employment Status:
☐ Employed ☐ Volunteer
☐ Student ☐ Retired
☐ Homemaker ☐ Unemployed
☐ Caregiver
Living Situation:
☐ Lives alone
☐ Assisted Living
☐ Institution (e.g., nursing home > 6 months)
☐ Lives with family
☐ Lives with friend/roommate
☐ Other _____
Years of Education:

Degree(s) Earned:

Independence in Occupational Behavior:
☐ Independent
☐ Needs assistance
☐ Totally dependent

My Environment	Environmental Impact			Value of Environment			
	problem	all right	well	not so important	important	extremely important	Priority
A place to live and take care of myself.							
A place where I can be productive (work, study, volunteer).							
The basic things I need to live and take care of myself.							
The things I need to be productive.							
People who support and encourage me.							
People who do things with me.							
Opportunities to do things I value and like.							
Places where I can go and enjoy myself.							

FIGURE A-1. Occupational Self-Assessment (OSA) Initial Evaluation Summary Form. This form may not be reproduced or used in any way without purchasing the manual. Occupational Self-Assessment Data Summary Sheet, from Baron, K., Kielhofner, G., Goldhammer, V., & Wolenski, J. (1998). *A user's manual for the Occupational Self-Assessment (OSA)* (Version 1.0). Chicago: University of Illinois at Chicago, reprinted with permission.

Method

This assessment is a paper-and-pencil self-report measure. A client can complete the self and environment rating forms on his or her own. However, it is best for you to be present when the client completes the self-report measure, to ensure that the client comprehends what is being asked and is responding appropriately. Moreover, even if the client completes the forms independently, you will need to meet with the client to discuss his or her therapy goals.

Psychometric Properties

An initial study with 202 adults (112 female; 90 male) of diverse language, culture, race, disability status, and age indicated the OSA is a valid assessment of levels of competence and environmental impact and of levels of importance clients ascribe to those factors.

Ordering Information

AOTA Products; P.O. Box 64949; Baltimore, MD 21264-4949; 1-800-SAY-AOTA for AOTA members; (301) 652-AOTA (2682) for nonmembers
[OSA information not from Henry (1998)]

THE CANADIAN OCCUPATIONAL PERFORMANCE MEASURE (COPM)

Purpose

The COPM (Law et al., 1998) was designed to measure a client's perceptions of his or her occupational performance over time.

Description

During an initial evaluation, the therapist interviews the client about his or her functioning in the areas of self-care, productivity, and leisure. (A specific set of interview questions has not been developed for the COPM.) The client is asked to identify any activities that are difficult for him or her to do in each area, and to indicate how important it is for him or her to be able to do those activities. Finally, the client is asked to identify his or her five most important problems, and to rate his or her performance and level of satisfaction in these activities (Figure A-2). The

APPENDIX A

importance of the activity to the client, the quality of the client's performance, and the client's level of satisfaction are all rated **by the client** using similar 10-point scales (1 = not important at all, not able to do it, and not satisfied at all; 10 = extremely important, able to do it extremely well, and extremely satisfied). The specific focus of the COPM on client-identified problems is intended to facilitate collaborative goal setting between the therapist and client. At a re-evaluation, the client is again asked to rate his or her performance and satisfaction relative to the problem areas identified in the initial evaluation. By doing this, changes in the client's perceptions over time can be detected (Law et al., 1998).

Method

This assessment is a client-centered semi-structured interview.

Psychometric Properties

In a study of 27 older adults with a variety of physical disabilities, test–retest reliability coefficients for Performance and Satisfaction scores were .63 and .84 respectively. A more recent study found test–retest reliability coefficients for Performance and Satisfaction scores of 0.80 and 0.89 respectively (Law, et al., 1998). Studies have also suggested that the COPM ratings are a valid indicator of clients' perceptions of the occupational performance. The COPM has also been found to be sensitive to changes in clients' performance and satisfaction ratings following occupational therapy and other rehabilitative interventions (Law, et al., 1998).

Ordering Information

Outside the United States, contact: Canadian Association of Occupational Therapists; CTTC Building, Suite 3400; 1125 Colonel Bay Drive;

Initial Assessment:			**Reassessment:**	
OCCUPATIONAL PERFORMANCE PROBLEMS:	PERFORMANCE 1	SATISFACTION 1	PERFORMANCE 1	SATISFACTION 1
1. ______				
2. ______				
3. ______				
4. ______				
5. ______				

FIGURE A-2. Part of Canadian Occupational Performance Measure (COPM) Form. From Canadian Occupational Performance Measure, 3rd edition, 1998, reprinted with permission.

Ottawa. ON KIS 5RI; Telephone: (800) 434-2268 or (613) 523-2268
x232; FAX: (613) 523-2552

In the United States, contact: AOTA Products; P.O. Box 64949; Baltimore, MD 21264-4949; 1-800-SAY-AOTA for AOTA members; (301)
652-AOTA (2682) for nonmembers

THE OCCUPATIONAL QUESTIONNAIRE (OQ)

Purpose

The Occupational Questionnaire (OQ) (Smith, Kielhofner, & Watts,
1986) was designed to provide information about clients' time use patterns and feelings about time use.

Description

The OQ is a paper-and-pencil measure that gathers data on time use
patterns and feelings about time use. In completing the OQ, the person indicates his or her main activity during each half hour of a typical day, and classifies each activity as either school, work, activity of
daily living (ADL), recreation, or rest. The person then rates each activity using a 5-point Likert-type scale, indicating how well he or she
does the activity (competence), how important the activity is (value),
and how enjoyable the activity is (enjoyment). The OQ is based on
Model of Human Occupation (MOHO) constructs.

Method

This assessment is a paper-and-pencil self-report measure. A client
can complete the checklist on his or her own. However, it is best for
you to be present when the client completes the self-report measure,
to ensure that the client comprehends what is being asked and is responding appropriately.

Psychometric Properties

In a test–retest reliability study of 20 elderly adults, 68% of a typical day's
activities reported during the first administration were again reported
during the same time period of the second administration. Agreement
on activity categorization and feelings of competence, value, and enjoyment was also high. A study of concurrent validity using the Household
Work Study Diary yielded high agreement in configuration of activities
and in how subjects' classified activities (Smith et al., 1986).

APPENDIX A

Ordering Information

Model of Human Occupation Clearinghouse: www.uic.edu/hsc/acad/cahp/OT/MOHOC/

THE ROLE CHECKLIST

Purpose

The Role Checklist (Oakley, Kielhofner, Barris, & Reichler, 1986) was designed to assess clients' values and intentions to perform their life roles.

Description

The Role Checklist (Oakley et al., 1986) is a two part inventory of ten occupational roles, including worker, student, family member, homemaker, caregiver, volunteer, and hobbyist. The first part of the Role Checklist examines a client's past, present, and future intentions related to performance of each role. The second part examines the value assigned to each role by the client.

Method

This assessment is a paper-and-pencil self-report measure. A client can complete the checklist on his or her own. However, it is best for you to be present when the client completes the self-report measure, to ensure that the client comprehends what is being asked and is responding appropriately.

Psychometric Properties

Studies have indicated that the Role Checklist has good test–retest reliability (Barris, Oakley, & Kielhofner, 1988) and is valid (Barris, Dickie, & Baron, 1988; Ebb et al., 1989; Smyntek, Barris, & Kielhofner, 1985).

Ordering Information

Contact: Fran Oakley, MS, OTR, FAOTA; National Institutes of Health; Building 10, Room 6s235; 10 Center Drive MSC 1604; Bethesda, MD 20892-1604; FAX: (301) 480-0669

APPENDIX

B

BASIC AND INSTRUMENTAL ACTIVITY OF DAILY LIVING ASSESSMENTS

ASSESSMENTS OF BASIC AND INSTRUMENTAL ACTIVITIES OF DAILY LIVING

Kohlman Evaluation of Living Skills (KELS)

Purpose. The KELS (McGourty, 1979, 1988) was designed to aid in discharge planning for clients with psychiatric diagnoses. It evaluates the ability to live independently and safely in the community and has also been used with geriatric clients and those with mental retardation, brain injury, and cognitive impairment.

Description. The 18 tasks included on the KELS are grouped into 5 categories: self-care, safety and health, money management, transportation and telephone, and work and leisure. Hence, the tasks span all occupational areas. Task performance is scored as 0, signifying independent and 1 or 1/2 signifying needs assistance. Independence means safe and healthy performance without the assistance of others. Assistance in six or more tasks is indicative of a need for a supportive living situation. Information about impairments influencing clients' performance, such as attention span, visual figure-ground, and com-

---

With the exception of ordering information, unless otherwise noted, the information in this appendix has been modified and reprinted with permission from: Rogers, J. C. & Holm, M. B. (1998). Evaluation of Activities of Daily Living (ADL) and home management. In M. E. Neistadt & E. B. Crepeau (Eds.), *Willard & Spackman's occupational therapy* (pp. 185–208). Philadelphia: Lippincott.

prehension, is included in a summary note. The KELS can be administered and scored in 30 to 45 minutes.

Method. The KELS combines interview and performance-based methods and tends to emphasis the knowledge-component of tasks.

Psychometric Properties. Percent rater agreement ranged from 74–94% in one study (Ilika & Hoffman, 1981a) and 84–94% in another (Tateichi, as cited in McGourty, 1988). The higher scores of residents of sheltered living situations compared to individuals living independently in the community were used to establish construct validity (Tateichi, as cited in McGourty, 1988). Evidence of concurrent validity was obtained from correlations between scores on the KELS and Bay Area Functional Performance Evaluation ($r = -0.84$; $p < .0001$) and the Global Assessment Scale (between $r = .78$ and $.89$; $p < .0001$) in samples of inpatient mental health clients (Ilika & Hoffman, 1981b; Kaufman, 1982). The results of predictive validity studies were inconclusive (McGourty, 1988; Morrow, as cited in McGourty, 1988).

Ordering Information. AOTA Products; P.O. Box 64949; Baltimore, MD 21264-4949; 1-800-SAY-AOTA for AOTA members; (301) 652-AOTA (2682) for nonmembers

Milwaukee Evaluation of Daily Living Skills (MEDLS)

Purpose. The MEDLS (Leonardelli, 1988a, b) was designed to establish baseline behaviors necessary to develop treatment objectives and guide intervention in regard to daily living skills for clients with chronic mental health problems.

Description. The MEDLS consists of 20 subtests covering the following: communication, personal care, clothing care, safety in the home and community, money management, personal health care, medication management, telephone use, transportation usage, and time awareness. The subtests can be administered individually or in combination. A screening form is used to ascertain the specific items to be examined for each client. The screening form can be employed as a tool for obtaining information from clients and their families, the health care team, and the medical record. Each subtest is scored according to the number of skills completed for that task. No summary score is calculated for the MEDLS because the administration of subtests varies from client to client. Subtests have a specified time for completion and when this time is exceeded, the practitioner makes a clinical judgment about the cause of the delay (e.g., comprehension, motivation).

Method. For testing, some activities are performed (e.g., dressing), others are simulated (e.g., bathing), and others are described (e.g., transportation).

Psychometric Properties. Interrater reliability coefficients for most subtests were above $r = .80$. Content validity is based on the literature and other similar instruments (Leonardelli, 1988a).

Ordering Information. Available in: Leonardelli, C. A. (1988a). *The Milwaukee Evaluation of Daily Living Skills.* Thorofare, NJ: SLACK, Inc. [SLACK Inc.; 6900 Grove Road; Thorofare, NJ 08086; 1-800-257-8290; FAX (609) 853-5991; www.slackinc.com]

Performance Assessment of Self-care Skills, Version 3.1 (PASS)

Purpose. The PASS (Rogers & Holm, 1989, 1994) was designed to evaluate the independent living skills of adults. It is a criterion-referenced instrument. It has been used with healthy, older adults as well as those with osteoarthritis, dementia, depression, cardiopulmonary disease, schizophrenia, bipolar affective disorder, mental retardation, and low vision. It can be used to assess baseline status and change over time following intervention or age-associated or disease-related changes. Further, it provides data useful for planning intervention or the support needed at discharge.

Description. The 26 items included on the PASS encompass functional mobility, personal care, **and** home management. For each task, the PASS yields three summary scores: independence, safety, and outcome. Each of these measurement parameters is rated on a 4-point ordinal scale with 0 representing dysfunction and 3 representing function. Independence ratings are applied to subtasks (i.e., lower self to tub bottom) rather than a task as a whole (i.e., tub transfer). This procedure enables the practitioner to identify the specific point or points in a task sequence where breakdown occurs. Further, the number and types of assists necessary for safe and adequate task performance are recorded, thus furnishing information useful for planning intervention, including supportive services. There are two protocols for the PASS—one for use in the home and the other for use in a client's living situation. The two protocols are identical in terms of the tasks included and the performance criteria. However, in the home, clients use their own task materials.

Method. The PASS is a performance-based observational tool.

Psychometric Properties. Percent agreement between two observers, whether done in the clinic or the home, ranged between 96% and 99%. Content validity of the PASS is based on four interview instruments for evaluating independent living skills—the Physical Self-Maintenance and Instrumental Self-Maintenance Scales (Lawton & Brody, 1969) the Activities of Daily Living Scale of the OARS Multidimensional Functional Assessment Questionnaire (Fillenbaum, 1988), the Comprehensive Assessment and Referral Evaluation (Gurland et al., 1977–78), and the Functional Assessment Questionnaire (Pfeffer et al., 1982). Construct validity is based on the performance of the instrument on groups with different medical and psychiatric diagnoses or level of acuity and on ADL and IADL categories. Thus, healthy adults score higher than those with depression and those with depression score higher than those with dementia. Inpatients with depression score lower at admission than at discharge but even at discharge they score lower than depressed outpatients. Outpatients with early dementia score lower in IADL than ADL skills.

Ordering Information. Contact: Joan Rogers & Margo Holm; Occupational Therapy Department; School of Health and Rehabilitation Sciences; University of Pittsburgh, 5012 Forbes Tower; Pittsburgh, PA 15260. Letter should include an explanation of why you want to use this instrument.

Routine Task Inventory-2 (RTI-2)

Purpose. The RTI-2 (Allen, Earhart, & Blue, 1992) is designed to establish the level of functional status and document change in status based on the Allen Cognitive Levels (ACL) (Allen, 1985, 1990). Thus, it relates cognitive impairment to task performance.

Description. Content of the RTI is based on the disability categories of the model of disablement proposed by the World Health Organization (1980). The 32 items encompass self-awareness disability (e.g., grooming, dressing, bathing), situational awareness disability (e.g., housekeeping, spending money, shopping), occupational role disability (e.g., planning/doing major role tasks, pacing and timing actions, speaking); and social role disability (e.g., communicating meaning, following instructions, caring for dependents). The behaviors that would be indicative of functioning at each of the six ACL levels are defined and described for each of the items. There are no standardized procedures or directions for administration or scoring. The practitioner matches descriptions or observations of performance with the operational definitions for each level of functioning. A 3-point to 6-point ordinal scale is used for each item, with lower scores indicating lower abilities and higher scores indicating higher abilities. For example, the highest score for grooming, which is a 5, means that clients can initiate and complete grooming without assistance; the lowest score for the same item, which is a 3, means that clients ignore personal appearance and may not cooperate with caregiving actions. For less complex behaviors in the self-awareness and situational awareness categories, the ACL levels defined for scoring range from 1 to 6 or 2 to 5; for more complex behaviors in the occupational and social role categories, the lowest ACL level defined for scoring is level 3 and the highest is level 6. The RTI-2 can be administered in either a clinic or a home setting.

Method. The RTI may be rated through observing or questioning, and clients or proxies may be respondents. Self-report is not recommended for clients at ACL levels 1 through 4.

Psychometric Properties. Interrater reliability ($r = 0.98$), test-retest reliability ($r = 0.91$), and internal consistency ($r = 0.94$) were established on the original version of the instrument. Evidence of validity was obtained from correlating RTI scores with those on the Mini-Mental State Examination. The obtained correlation of $r_s = .61$ supported the relationship between functional decline and cognitive impairment (Allen, Kehrberg, & Burns, 1992). Correlations between the RTI and the ACL levels were calculated as $r_s = 0.54$ to 0.56 (Heimann, Allen, & Yerxa, 1989; Wilson, Allen, McCormack, & Burton, 1989).

Ordering Information. Available in: Allen, C. K., Earhart, C. A., & Blue, T. (1992). *Occupational therapy treatment goals for the physically and cognitively challenged.* Rockville, MD: American Occupational Therapy Association. [AOTA Products; P.O. Box 64949; Baltimore, MD 21264-4949; 1-800-SAY-AOTA for AOTA members; (301) 652-AOTA (2682) for nonmembers]

APPENDIX B

ASSESSMENTS OF BASIC ACTIVITIES OF DAILY LIVING

Árnadóttir OT-ADL Neurobehavioral Evaluation (A-ONE)

Purpose. The A-One (Árnadóttir, 1990) has a dual purpose: (a) to assess independence in selected ADL and the types of assistance needed to complete them and (b) to identify the types and severity of neurobehavioral impairment. These data are to be used to assist in setting goals and planning treatment. The A-One was designed for use with adults with central nervous system dysfunctions having cortical origin.

Description. Part 1 of the A-One encompasses the Functional Independence Scale and the Neurobehavioral Specific Impairment Scale. The former scale covers five ADL domains, namely, dressing, grooming and hygiene, transfer and mobility, feeding, and communication. The latter scale accompanies each of the ADL domains and includes 11 impairments (e.g., motor apraxia, ideational apraxia, perseveration), except when applied to feeding and communication where it is modified. The ADL and neurobehavioral impairments are rated on a 5-point ordinal scale, ranging from 0 to 4. The high point of the functional scale connotes independence and the ability to transfer the task to other situations while the low point connotes an inability to perform the task, that is, being totally dependent on assistance. The neurobehavioral scale ranges from no observed impairment to client needs maximum physical assistance related to severe neurobehavioral impairment. The intent of Part II of the A-One, the Neurobehavioral Scale Summary Sheet, is to assist practitioners in identifying the most likely lesion site for the identified neurobehavioral deficits. Part II is not meant to be a diagnostic tool but rather to foster understanding of the central nervous system deficit so that an appropriate intervention plan can be formulated. Completion of Part II is optional.

Method. Data for Part 1 are gathered through informal observation. Part II relies on the practitioner's clinical reasoning about the underlying cause or causes of task performance deficits.

Psychometric Properties. Interrater reliability for the Functional Independence Scale achieved a kappa coefficient of .83 and for the Neurobehavioral Specific Impairment Scale .86. Test-retest reliability for items in Part 1 with a one week interval was at least $r_s = .85$. Content validity of the A-One is based on literature reviews and expert judgment. In a sample of normal individuals no ADL disabilities or neurobehavioral impairments were evidenced. Individuals with cerebral vascular accident scored lower than normal individuals on both scales. The instrument appears to have the capability of detecting ADL improvement.

Ordering Information. Available in: Árnadóttir, G. (1990). *The brain and behavior: Assessing cortical dysfunction through tasks of daily living.* St. Louis: The C. V. Mosby Co. [Mosby, Inc.; 11830 Westline Industrial Drive; St. Louis, MO 63146-3318; 1-800-222-9570; www.mosby.com]

Functional Independence Measure (FIM)

Purpose. The FIM (UDSMR, 1993) measures disability associated with physical impairments. It is a part of the Uniform Data System for Medical Rehabilitation, and as such provides a mechanism for standardizing data collection nationwide for clients entering medical rehabilitation. The FIM was devised to provide a more comprehensive measure of disability than was previously available on functional assessments, such as the Barthel and the Index of ADL, by expanding functional mobility and personal self-care and including communication and cognitive function. It is not intended to provide a comprehensive disability evaluation covering all occupational areas.

Description. Eighteen critical tasks are included on the FIM. Of these, 13 have a motor emphasis and are related to self-care (i.e., feeding, grooming, bathing, dressing upper body, dressing lower body, toileting), sphincter control (i.e., bladder and bowel management), mobility (bed, chair, wheelchair, toilet, and tub or shower transfers) and locomotion (walk or wheelchair, stairs). The remaining five have a cognitive emphasis and involve communication (i.e., comprehension, expression) and social cognition (i.e., social interaction, problem solving, memory) (Linacre et al., 1994). The type and amount of assistance required to perform tasks is used to measure disability severity and care burden. Tasks are scored using a 7-point or 4-point scale. A score of 7 reflects complete independence; 6, modified independence which implies some delay, safety risk, or device usage; 5, supervision; 4, minimal assistance with clients exerting 75% plus effort; 3, moderate assistance with clients exerting 50% plus effort; 2, complete dependence with clients exerting 25% plus effort; and 1, total assistance with the subject exerting less than 24% effort. The 7-point scale converts to a 4-level on as follows: 4 = independence (#7); 3 = modified independence (#6); 2 = modified dependence (#5,4,3); and 1 = dependence (#2,1). The

APPENDIX B

potential for detecting change in disability is greater with the 7-point than the 4-point scale. The rationale underlying the rating scale is that the amount of assistance needed by clients to complete tasks is an index of the social and the economic costs of disability.

Method. The FIM requires observation of task performance and rating by a trained observers, who may be practitioners, clients, or family members. A telephone version is available (Jaworski, Kult, & Boynton, 1994).

Psychometric Properties. Using the 4-point scale, the intraclass correlation for total FIM scores was found to be .86 at admission and .88 at discharge from rehabilitation. The average kappa statistic for each of the 18 items was .54 (Hamilton et al., 1987). The FIM has been transformed from an ordinal to an interval scale through Rasch analysis and the structure of the motor and cognitive scales have been shown to be stable at admission and discharge (Linacre et al., 1994). This gives the FIM an advantage over other disability measures because it can be used more accurately to measure clinical change and for research purposes. FIM admission scores can predict discharge status and length of stay in rehabilitation, although predictive power varies with impairment type. Function in motor tasks emerged as a more important predictor of length of stay than function in cognitive tasks. Shorter stays were associated with greater cognitive capability for clients with traumatic brain injury and lesser cognitive capability for those with stroke and neurologic impairments (Heinemann et al., 1994).

Ordering Information. Uniform Data System for Medical Rehabilitation; University at Buffalo; 232 Parker Hall; 3435 Main Street; Buffalo, NY 14214-3007; (716) 829-2076; FAX: (716) 829-2080: e-mail: info@udsmr.org; www.udsmr.org

Klein-Bell Activities of Daily Living Scale (Klein-Bell)

Purpose. The Klein-Bell (Klein & Bell, 1979, 1982) was designed to measure ADL independence in children and adults. It is useful for determining current status, change in status, and the subtasks to focus on during intervention.

Description. The Klein-Bell has 170 items in six domains: dressing, mobility, elimination, bathing/hygiene, eating, and emergency communication. Task analysis was used to identify critical and observable subtasks in the tasks included in these domains. Each subtask is scored as able to perform, unable, or not applicable. An expert panel of rehabilitation professionals was used to establish subtask weights and weights of 1, 2, or 3 were assigned to each subtask. In weighing the items four factors were considered: its importance to health, its difficulty for a non-disabled person, the time required to perform it, and, the associated burden of caregiving. The total points achieved within each domain are added to give an overall independence score. These scores can range from 0 to 313, but are expressed as percentages of the total points possible.

Method. The Klein-Bell Scale is an observational instrument.

Psychometric Properties. Interrater agreement across all items was estimated as 92%. Evidence of predictive validity was obtained from correlations between Klein-Bell scores and the hours clients required assistance per week for a 5- to 10-month period following discharge (Klein & Bell, 1982). Use of the Klein-Bell to examine bathing training, suggests that it is capable of measuring change (Shillam, Beeman, & Loshin, 1983).

Ordering Information. HSCER Distribution; HSB T277 Box 357161; University of Washington; Seattle, WA 98195; FAX: (206) 543-8051; Phone: (206) 685-1186; e-mail: center@u.washington.edu

ASSESSMENTS OF INSTRUMENTAL ACTIVITIES OF DAILY LIVING

Assessment of Living Skills and Resources (ALSAR)

Purpose. The ALSAR (Williams et al., 1991) was developed to assess IADL as well as to identify needs, assign risk, and prioritize intervention. A unique feature of the instrument is the consideration of IADL skills in relation to the resources available to mitigate skill deficits. While skills are intrinsic to clients, and represent their ability to perform tasks or procure services, resources are extrinsic to clients, and represent human or technical, formal or informal supports for task accomplishment. Conceptually, IADL deficits must not be interpreted solely in terms of skills but rather from the perspective of the environmental resources available to compensate for these deficits. Thus, a client with arthritis who was unable to do laundry, housekeeping, or home maintenance would not be at risk if a sibling were available to do these tasks.

APPENDIX B

Description. The 11 IADL included on the ALSAR are: telephoning, reading, leisure task, medication management, money management, transportation, shopping, meal preparation, laundering, housekeeping, and home maintenance. For each task, skill is rated as independent, partially independent, or dependent and resources are rated as consistently available, inconsistently available, and not available or in use. The 3-point skill and resources scales range from a high of 0 to a low of 2. The skill and resources scores are combined to obtain a risk score for each IADL (Figure B-1). Risk is designated as low (combined

ASSESSMENT OF LIVING SKILLS AND RESOURCES (ALSAR)				
ALSAR TASKS	**SKILLS** (Individual accomplishes or procures task) Independent - 0 Partially Independent - 1 Dependent - 2 Record SKILL level	**TASK RISK SCORE** Combined Skill + Resource Level 3 or 4 = High 2 = Moderate 0 or 1 = Low		**RESOURCES** (Support for task completion extrinsic to individual) 0 - Consistently Available 1 - Inconsistently Available 2 - Not Available or in Use Record RESOURCE level
Telephoning	Locates phone numbers, dials, sends and receives information			Resources for telephoning
Reading	Reads and uses written information			Resources for reading
Leisure	Plans and performs satisfying leisure activities			Resources for satisfying leisure activities
Medication Management	Procures and takes medicine as ordered			Resources for managing medications
Money Management	Manages finances or procures financial services			Resources for managing finances
Transportation	Walks, drives, or procures rides			Resources for transportation
Shopping	Lists, selects, buys, orders, stores goods			Resources for shopping
Meal Preparation	Performs all aspects of meal preparation or procures meals			Resources for meal preparation
Laundering	Performs or procures all aspects of doing laundering			Resources for laundering
Housekeeping	Cleans own living space or procures housekeeping service			Resources for housekeeping
Home Maintenance	Performs or procures home maintenance			Resources for home maintenance

"R" SCORE ⬭ (sum of 11 TASK RISK SCORES)

Name: _____   Interviewer: _____

Date: _____   Information Source: _____

©1991 ALSAR-Revised Format. T.J.K. Drinka; J.H. Williams; M. Schram; J. Farrell-Holtan; R. Euhardy: VAMC, Madison, WI 53705

FIGURE B-1. Assessment of Living Skills and Resources (ALSAR) Evaluation Form. Reprinted with permission from Madison Geriatric Research, Education and Clinical Center; William S. Memorial Veteran's Hospital, with permission.

score of 0 or 1), moderate (combined score of 3), or high (combined score of 4). The risk score assists in setting priorities for intervention.

Method. The ALSAR is an interview measure and questions are provided to assist in data gathering.

Psychometric Properties. Internal consistency using Cronbach's alpha was calculated as .91. Interrater percent agreement ranged from 72% to 94% for skills and 78% to 100% for resources. Content validity of the ALSAR is based on the expert judgment of geriatric practitioners from occupational and physical therapy and social work. Evidence of criterion related validity was obtained from significant correlations between the risk score and the following changes at 6-month follow-up: move to a more structured living situation; move to a more supportive living situation, nursing home placement, hospitalization, and death. The risk score also correlated with measures of mental status and ADL status but not with depression and caregiver burden.

Ordering Information. Contact: Madison Geriatric Research, Education and Clinical Center; William S. Middleton Memorial Veteran's Hospital; 2500 Overlook Terrace; Madison, WI 53705; (608) 262-7089, for a master copy of the ALSAR; two 1/2″ videotapes also available: "Overview of IADL Assessment" and "Administration of the ALSAR."

Assessment of Motor and Process Skills (AMPS)

Purpose. The AMPS (Fisher, 1994) is used to examine the relationship between motor and process skills and task performance, to establish current level of task competence, and to predict performance in IADL. It is useful for treatment planning. It has been used with children, adolescents, and adults with a variety of underlying impairments.

Description. The AMPS consists of 56 calibrated tasks, such as sweep the floor, repot a plant, and change sheets on a bed. Tasks are rated on 16 motor skills (e.g., reaches, lifts, paces) and 20 process skills (initiates, searches, adjusts). Each motor and process skill item is rated on a 4-point ordinal score ranging from 1, which signifies that the deficit is severe enough to result in damage, danger, or task breakdown to 4, which signifies that there is no evidence of a deficit that impacts performance, that is, competence. AMPS items scores are then transformed from ordinal to an interval scale with a many-faceted Rasch analysis program (Linacre, 1989), which allows them to be adjusted based on rater leniency and task difficulty. This analysis also makes it possible to predict a client's performance on the other calibrated task (Doble, Fisk, Ritvo, & Murray, 1994). The AMPS takes 30 to 60 minutes to administer.

Method. Clients' normal routines are identified through interview. Subsequently, the practitioner suggestions five or six tasks for clients to perform, asks them to select several from these options, and observes and rates their performance.

Psychometric Properties. Of the 300 trained raters, 95% have achieved Rasch goodness-of-fit statistics that indicate adequate inter-rater reliability (Doble et al., 1994). For tasks to be considered valid, they must fit a preestablished Rasch measurement model. The AMPS has undergone extensive validity testing, including comparisons between settings (Nygård, Bernspång, Fisher, & Winblad, 1994) and across cultures (Fisher, Liu, Velozo, & Pan, 1992).

Ordering Information. Special training is required for the use of this instrument. For more information, contact:
Colorado State University; Occupational Therapy Building; AMPS Project; Fort Collins, CO 80523

Rabideau Kitchen Evaluation-Revised (RKE-R)

Purpose. The RKE-R (Neistadt, 1992) was designed to evaluate the the functional sequencing ability of adults with TBI (Neistadt, 1992; Rabideau, 1986). It can be used to help establish intervention goals and to track client change over time.

Description. The RKE-R requires subjects to prepare a simple meal— a cold sandwich with two fillings and a hot instant beverage. On the evaluation form, the sandwich and beverage tasks are broken down into 40 component steps. These steps are listed in the order they are most commonly performed, but subjects are not required to follow this exact order. Each component step on the evaluation form is scored according to the following scale:

0 = Subject requires no assistance. He/she initiates and performs the component step independently.

1 = Subject requires one verbal cue or instruction to perform the component step.

2 = Subject requires more than one verbal cue or instruction to perform the component step.

3 = Subject is unable to perform the component step and requires direct intervention from the evaluator to complete the step.

The minimum possible score is zero and indicates total independence. The maximum possible score is 120 and indicated a need for physical assistance with all steps of the sandwich and beverage tasks.

Method. The RKE-R is an observational tool.

Psychometric Properties. The RKE-R has a test-retest coefficient of 0.80 and an interrater agreement of 86% (Neistadt, 1992). The evaluation has content validity since it was developed from the occupational therapy literature and subject to expert review. The RKE-R also has criterion-related validity as demonstrated by a significant Pearson correlation coefficient between scores on the RKE-R, a functional test of sequencing, and WAIS-R Block Design, which also taps sequencing ($r = -0.60$; $p = 0.0002$). The correlation was negative because good performance is indicated by low scores on the RKE-R and high scores on the WAIS-R Block Design test (Neistadt, 1992).

Ordering Information. Contact: Maureen E. Neistadt; Occupational Therapy Department; School of Health and Human Services; University of New Hampshire; Hewitt Hall; 4 Library Way; Durham, NH 03824-3563; e-mail: maureenn@cisunix.unh.edu
[RKE-R information not from Roger & Holm (1998).]

Satisfaction With Performance Scaled Questionnaire (SPSQ)

Purpose. The SPSQ (Yerxa, Burnett-Beaulieu, Stocking, & Azen, 1988) was designed to operationalize satisfaction experienced in the performance of independent living skills. Satisfaction is defined as perceived pleasure or contentment. The SPSQ is useful for identifying intervention goals for community-based persons with disabilities as areas of low satisfaction may be targeted for independent living skills training.

Description. The SPSQ contains two subscales involving independent living skills. Subscale I, Home Management, contains 24 items relevant to this occupational area. Typical items are: scrape/stack dishes, use stove top elements, clean bathtub/shower, handle a milk carton, and stir against resistance in a bowl. Subscale II, is titled Social/Community, and contains 22 items. Some of these items are typically included under home management (e.g., pay bill and balance account, budget your income), while others are more oriented toward interpersonal, educational, vocational, and leisure skills. Each item is scored on a 5-point scale using the percentage of time over the past six months that clients felt satisfied with their performance as the reference point. The percentage scale ranges from all (100%) of the time to none (0%) of the time.

Method. The SPSQ is a self-report questionnaire.

Psychometric Properties. Split-half reliability coefficients were 0.97 and 0.93 for the Home Management and Social/Community Problem Solving scales respectively. Evidence suggestive of construct validity was obtained from a small study in which clients with spinal cord injury scored lower than nondisabled subjects on the Home Management and Social/Community scales.

Ordering Information. Available in: Yerxa, E. J., Burnett-Beaulieu, S., Stocking, S., & Azen, S. P. (1988). Development of the satisfaction with scaled performance questionnaire (SPSQ). *American Journal of Occupational Therapy, 42,* 215–22.

The Worker Role Interview (WRI)

Purpose. The WRI was designed to gather data on psychosocial and environmental factors related to work, for injured workers (Velozo, Kielhofner, & Fisher, 1992). While the WRI was originally developed for use with individuals with physical disabilities, it has recently been adapted for use with individuals with psychiatric disorders (Handelsman, 1994).

Description. The WRI is comprised of a set of 28 recommended questions and an accompanying 17-item rating scale, and was developed to be compatible with the Model of Human Occupation (MOHO). The items form six subscales that reflect the worker's sense of personal causation, values, interests, roles and habits related to work, as well as the influence of the environment. Each of the 17 items is rated using a 4-point scale (4 = strongly supports client returning to job; 1 = strongly interferes with client returning to job).

Method. The WRI is a semi-structured interview.

Psychometric Properties. Biernacki (1993) found good interrater and test-retest reliability for the WRI studies of adults with upper extremity injuries.

Ordering Information. AOTA Products; P.O. Box 64949; Baltimore, MD 21264-4949; 1-800-SAY-AOTA for AOTA members; (301) 652-AOTA (2682) for nonmembers
[Information on the WRI modified and reprinted, with permission, from Henry, A. (1998). The interview process in occupational therapy. In M. E. Neistadt & E. B. Crepeau (Eds.), *Willard & Spackman's Occupational Therapy* (pp. 155–168). Philadelphia: Lippincott.]

APPENDIX

C

SOMATIC SENSORY EVALUATION PROCEDURES

The information in this appendix has been modified and reprinted with permission from: Kohlmeyer, K. (1998). Evaluation of sensory and neuromuscular performance components. In M.E. Neistadt & E.B. Crepeau (Eds.), *Willard & Spackman's occupational therapy* (9th ed.) (pp. 223–260). Philadelphia: Lippincott.

APPENDIX C

GENERAL METHODOLOGY PRINCIPLES

The following principles apply to all somatic sensation testing.

1) Explain the procedure to the client. Ask for feedback/questions.
2) Give instructions when the client's eyes are not occluded. Demonstrate on non-involved extremity if there is one.
3) Test non-affected area to
   a) determine client's understanding
   b) establish what is normal for that individual
4) Occlude client's vision (e.g., via a manila folder, screen, eyes closed). Have client open eyes in between tests to avoid dizziness or disorientation.
5) Apply stimuli
   a) proximal to distal.
   b) randomly interspersed with non-presentation trials.
   c) on dorsal and ventral surfaces.
6) If client cannot respond verbally, he or she can point to a duplicate stimulus or picture or replicate movement if appropriate.
7) Enter results on form, date, and sign.

8) Scoring, definitions, and recording methods should be consistent (Smith, 1993; Bentzel, 1995)

The environment should be conducive to testing. The client should understand the general purpose and specific procedure and be able to actively participate and communicate responses. Specific testing procedures for primary and discriminative somatic sensation are delineated below.

PRIMARY SOMATIC SYSTEM

1. *Light touch* (ability to feel light touch)
   Stimulus: Light touch on a small area of the client's skin with a cotton swab, eraser tip or therapist's fingertip.
   Response: Client gives an indication when stimulus is felt via "now," "yes," describe or point to location (Bentzel, 1995; Dunn, 1991; Pedretti, 1996c).
   Fine gradations of light touch can be evaluated using the Semmes-Weinstein Calibrated Monofilament Test. This test controls the amount of force applied to the client's hand via a calibrated, hand-held instrument. This type of evaluation is particularly important for clients with peripheral nerve involvement. The Semmes-Weinstein Monofilament Test has intra/inter-instrument and intra/interrater reliability as well as administration and interpretation guidelines (Fess, 1993).
2. *Pain* (ability to feel pain)
   Stimulus: Safety pin with one sharp, one blunt end. Therapist applies mixed sharp and dull stimuli randomly with same degree of pressure.
   Response: Client gives an indication when and which stimulus is felt via "sharp" or "dull."
   Note. Pin should be cleaned with an alcohol swab before and after testing. (Bentzel, 1995; Dunn, 1991; Pedretti, 1996c).
3. *Temperature* (ability to distinguish variations in temperature)
   Stimulus: Capped test tubes (metal conduct better than glass); one filled with ice water, one with hot tap water tolerable to normal touch. Randomly alternate use of each stimulus, keeping on body surface long enough to allow a temperature change to occur on the skin (approx. 1 second).
   Response: Client gives an indication which stimulus is felt via "hot" or "cold" to each stimulus (Bentzel, 1995; Dunn, 1991; Pedretti, 1996c).

DISCRIMINATIVE SOMATIC SYSTEM

1. *Tactile localization* (ability to localize touch)

   Stimulus: Therapist touches client's skin with eraser tip or fingertip. Stimulus intensity and duration significantly influence accuracy of response.

   Response: After each stimulus, client opens eyes and places finger/describes area touched (Bentzel, 1995).

2. *Two-point discrimination* (ability to perceive two distinct stimuli when touched with two stimuli simultaneously)

   Stimulus: Aesthesiometer, Boley Gauge, or paper clip. Two points are applied simultaneously along the longitudinal axis in the center of the zone to be tested, with equal light pressure to the palmar surface of the forearm, hand, and fingers. Therapist adjusts the distance between the double stimuli during testing to identify the amount of distance needed between the two stimuli before the client perceives that two stimuli are present. One-point application trials are interspersed with test trials.

   Response: Client identifies stimulus via "one" or "two" points. A score is recorded for each skin area examined. Several normative values exist for distance between the double stimuli felt (Bentzel, 1995; Dunn, 1991).

3. *Stereognosis* (ability to identify objects tactually)

   Stimulus: Common object is placed in individual's hand (i.e. pen, key, quarter, cotton ball). Individual is asked to manipulate and identify the object. Test is not appropriate if client is not able to manipulate object on own.

   Response: Client names object(s) as it is identified, describes properties if unable to name object, or points to a choice via a photograph or display of identical objects (Bentzel, 1995; Dunn, 1991; Pedretti, 1996c).

4. *Proprioception* (ability to identify limb position in space without vision)

   Stimulus: Therapist holds body part being tested laterally to avoid cutaneous input and slowly, passively positions the joint being tested. Joints are tested singly and in combination.

   Response: Client is asked to reproduce the position with the opposite extremity. If unable to copy limb position, may give verbal response such as "up," "down," use a gesture or by pointing to directional arrows (Bentzel, 1995; Dunn, 1991; Pedretti, 1996c).

5. *Kinesthesia* (movement sense)

   Stimulus: Therapist holds body part being tested laterally to reduce tactile input and moves the joint up or down. Level of detec-

APPENDIX C

tion of kinesthesia is influenced by velocity. It is easier to detect brisk movement.

Response: After each stimulus, the client indicates in which direction the body part was moved (Pedretti, 1996c).

RECORDING RESULTS

Recorded results should be specific enough to enable future comparison of progress and to communicate useful information to others. Sensation could be recorded as intact, impaired, or absent. Recording options include graphic methods, diagrams, peripheral nerve distribution, dermatome distribution, and/or the number correct/the number of trials (such as stereognosis). Figures C-1, C-2, and 2-29 display recording sample forms.

Pain/Temp			Proprioception			Two Point Discrimination N: .3-.6 cm P: .6-1.2 cm S: 1.2....cm		
L		R	L		R			
C 4			Shoulder					
C 5			Elbow					
C 6			Wrist			L		R
C 7			Hand			C 6		
C 8						C 7		
T 1						C 8		

Note. N=no apparent deficit; P=partial deficit; S=severe deficit; NE=not examined.

FIGURE C-1. Sensory Record for Pain/Temperature and Two-point Discrimination by Dermatome and for Proprioception by Joint. Reprinted with permission from the Rehabilitation Institute of Chicago. (Figure 16-2, p. 229 in Willard & Spackman, 9th edition).

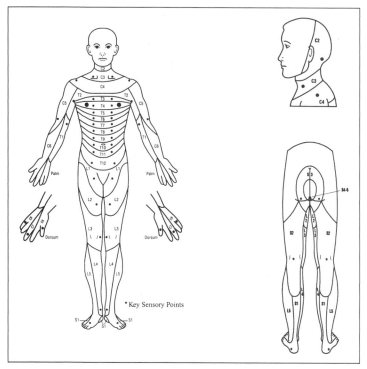

FIGURE C-2. Dermatome Chart for Recording Results of Sensory Testing. Reprinted with permission from the American Spinal Injury Association.

INTERPRETING RESULTS

Therapists must be alert to the influence of cognitive, perceptual, psychosocial, and motor deficits on sensory performance. Some clients may not be able to attend to or appreciate the abstract nature of tests used to evaluate sensation. They may have difficulty comprehending instructions, may guess at responses or find the procedure irrelevant and not fully participate. It is important to ask the client to describe (if able) what they feel. Observe during functional activities. Do they use proper force when grasping an object? Do they acknowledge or feel uncomfortable when touched? Are they aware of the position of their extremities when getting dressed? Do they drop items when not looking directly at the item? If sensation appears to be a contributing source to performance problems, accurately identify which deficits contribute to the problems. Educate the client, team members, and caregivers to the deficits and potential functional ramifications, such as safety issues, compensatory techniques, and environmental adaptations to facilitate sensory awareness and processing (Dunn, 1991; Okkema, 1993a).

APPENDIX C

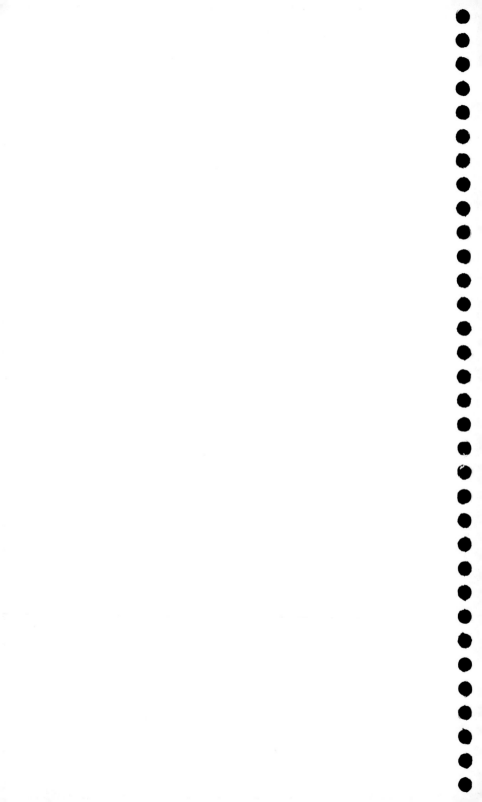

COGNITIVE/PERCEPTUAL ASSESSMENTS

BEHAVIORAL INATTENTION TEST (BIT)

Purpose

The BIT (Wilson, Cockburn, & Baddeley, 1987) was designed to evaluate visuo-spatial inattention.

Description

The BIT has six paper-and-pencil subtests and nine behavioral subtests. The paper and pencil tests include: line crossing, letter cancellation, star cancellation, figure and shape copying, line bisection, and representational drawing. The behavioral tests include: picture scanning, telephone dialing, menu reading, article reading, telling and setting the time, coin sorting, address and sentence copying, map navigation, and card sorting. The score for each subtest is the number of omissions. The number of omissions on the paper-and-pencil subtests yields a total score that determines the presence of unilateral spatial inattention. The performance on the behavioral subtests indicates how the inattention is affecting day-to-day activities (Zoltan, 1996).

Method

This is a therapist-administered test.

Psychometric Properties

Studies of the BIT have established an interrater reliability of 0.99 ($p = 0.001$), parallel form reliability between two test versions of 0.91 ($p = 0.001$), and test-retest reliability of 0.99 ($p = 0.001$). Construct validity is supported by the high correlation found between scores on the

BIT paper-and-pencil subtests which represent conventional tests of inattention, and the behavioral subtests ($r = 0.92$; p $= 0.001$) (Zoltan, 1996). Construct and predictive validity was further supported by a study comparing the performance of adults with stroke on three measures: the BIT, performance tasks, and an ADL checklist. Seven of the nine behavioral tests differentiated between those with and those without inattention and six of the nine behavioral subtests correlated significantly with similar performance on ADL checklist items (Hartman-Maeir & Katz, 1995).

Ordering Information

Western Psychological Services; Publishers and Distributors; 12031 Wilshire Boulevard; Los Angeles, CA 90025-1251; 1-800-648-8857; FAX: (310) 478-2061; www.wpspublish.com

CONTEXTUAL MEMORY TEST (CMT)

Purpose

The CMT (Toglia, 1993) was designed to "objectively measure awareness and strategy use in adults with memory impairment and/or screen for memory impairment which may require further testing" (Zoltan, 1996, p. 137).

Description

Through a combination of interview, task performance, and response to visual stimuli, the test items cover the following areas: awareness of memory capacity, recall of line drawn objects (immediate and delayed), and strategy use. The test has clients predict their memory skills before task performance, and estimate their memory skills following task performance. Immediate, delayed, and total recall raw scores are converted to standard scores. Prediction and estimation scores can also be generated. Data related to strategy use include the effect of context, total strategy use, and the order of recall (Zoltan, 1996).

Psychometric Properties

Partial test–retest reliability in one study ranged from 0.74 to 0.87 for the control group and from 0.85 to 0.94 for the group with brain injury. Correlations of 0.80–0.84 between the CMT and the Rivermead Behavioral Memory Test established concurrent validity for the CMT (Zoltan, 1996).

Ordering Information

Therapy Skill Builders; 555 Academic Court; San Antonio, TX 78204-2498; 1-800-211-8378; FAX: 1-800-232-1223; TDD 1-800-723-1318; www.hbtpc.com

LOWENSTEIN OCCUPATIONAL THERAPY COGNITIVE ASSESSMENT (LOTCA)

Purpose

The LOTCA (Itzkovitch, Elazar, Averbuch, & Katz, 1990) was designed as a concise battery of tests to measure cognitive and perceptual abilities. It can provide a baseline for intervention planning and serve as a measure of client change.

Description

There are 20 subtests grouped into 4 categories: orientation, perception, visuomotor organization, and thinking operations. The three categorization tests in the thinking operations category are scored on a scale of 1 (unable to perform) to 5 (good performance; can perform and verbalize criterion). All other tests are scored on a scale of 1 (unable to perform) to 4 (good performance). Attention and concentration are observed throughout the testing and scored on a scale of 1 (very short attention span; client cannot concentrate more than 5 minutes and needs continuous repetitions of instructions) to 4 (no attention or concentration problems). The LOTCA can be administered and scored in 30–45 minutes with some clients; others may need more time.

Method

The LOTCA is a therapist-administered battery.

Psychometric Properties

Normative scores are available for adults aged 20–70 years, based on samples of 20 adults with cranio-cerebral injury (CCI), 28 adults with stroke, and 55 healthy elders. Percent rater agreement on the subtests ranged from 86% to 100% in one study; interrater reliability ranged from 0.82 to 0.97 in another study (Itzkovitch, Elazar, Averbuch, & Katz, 1990). High internal consistency coefficients were found for per-

APPENDIX D

ception (0.87), visuomotor organization (0.95), and thinking operations (0.85) areas of the battery; this data support the structure of the battery. Construct validity was established by the significantly higher scores of healthy elders compared to individuals with brain injury. Evidence of concurrent validity was obtained from correlations between scores on the LOTCA visuomotor organization area and the Block Design subtest of the Wechsler Adult Intelligence Scale (WAIS) for adults with CCI, with timed ($r = 0.68$) and untimed ($r = 0.77$) versions of the WAIS Block Design test (Itzkovitch, Elazar, Averbuch, & Katz, 1990).

Ordering Information

North Coast Medical; 18305 Sutter Boulevard; Morgan Hill, CA 95037-2845; 1-800-821-9319; Toll Free FAX: (877) 213-9300; www.ncmedical.com

Sammons Preston; P.O. Box 5071; Bolingbrook, IL 60440-5071; 1-800-323-5547; FAX: 1-800-547-4333; e-mail: sp@sammonspreston.com

Smith Nephew; One Quality Drive, P.O. Box 1005; Germantown, WI 53022-8205 USA; 1-800-558-8633; FAX: 1-800-545-7758; www.easy-living.com

LOWENSTEIN OCCUPATIONAL THERAPY COGNITIVE ASSESSMENT FOR GERIATRIC POPULATION (LOTCA-G)

Purpose

The LOTCA-G (Elazar, Itzkovitch, , & Katz, 1996) was designed as a concise battery of tests to measure cognitive and perceptual abilities for older adults. Changes were made in this version of the test to account for the sensory problems and slowed processing experienced by many older adults (e.g., enlarged items to reduce vision or motor coordination difficulties). The LOTCA-G can provide a baseline for intervention planning and serve as a measure of client change.

Description

There are 19 subtests grouped into 5 categories: orientation, memory, perception, visuomotor organization, and thinking operations. The answers to each of the four questions in the orientation subtests are scored either 1 (no correct answer or one correct answer by multiple choice) or 2 (spontaneous, correct answer). All other tests are scored on a scale of 1 (poor performance) to 4 (good performance). Exact performance criteria for each point on the scale are given for each subtest. Attention and concentration are observed throughout the testing and scored on a scale of 1 (very short attention span; client cannot concentrate more than 5 minutes and needs continuous repetitions of instructions) to 4 (no attention or concentration problems). The LOTCA-G can be administered and scored in 30–45 minutes.

Method

The LOTCA-G is a therapist-administered battery.

Psychometric Properties

Normative scores are available for adults aged 20 to 91 years, based on samples of 33 adults with stroke and 43 healthy elders. Percent rater agreement was 90% in one study (Elazar, Itzkovitch, , & Katz, 1996). Construct validity was established by the significantly higher scores of healthy elders compared to individuals with brain injury.

Ordering Information

North Coast Medical; 18305 Sutter Boulevard; Morgan Hill, CA 95037-2845; 1-800-821-9319; Toll Free FAX: (877) 213-9300; www. ncmedical.com

Sammons Preston; P.O. Box 5071; Bolingbrook, IL 60440-5071; 1-800-323-5547; FAX: 1-800-547-4333; e-mail: sp@sammonspreston.com

Smith Nephew; One Quality Drive, P.O. Box 1005; Germantown, WI 53022-8205 USA; 1-800-558-8633; FAX: 1-800-545-7758; www.easy-living.com

MINI-MENTAL STATE (MMS)

Purpose

The MMS (Folstein, Folstein, & McHugh, 1975) was designed to evaluate cognitive aspects of mental function.

Description

The MMS includes 11 questions that cover the areas of orientation, memory registration, attention and calculation, recall, and language. It can be administered in 5–10 minutes. The questions are divided into two sections. The questions in sections one (orientation, memory, attention

APPENDIX D

and calculation, and recall) require verbal responses only, for a maximum score of 21. The questions in the second part (language) require clients to name, follow verbal and written commands, write a sentence spontaneously, and copy a complex polygon, for a maximu score of 9.

Method

The MMS is a therapist administered interview.

Psychometric Properties

Normative data are available for 137 adults with diagnoses of dementia, affective disorder, depressed type, affective disorder, manic type, schizophrenia, personality disorder with substance abuse, and neurosis. Studies on the MMS have demonstrated a test–retest reliability of 0.887 for two administrations of the test separated by 24 hours. Interrater reliability was 0.827. Construct validity was established by the fact that the MMS separated three diagnostic groups from one another and from a healthy group. When clients were retested after treatment, the MMS also showed no significant change for clients with dementia, a small but significant change for clients with depression, and a large and significant change for clients with depression with symptoms of cognitive difficulty. Concurrent validity was established by significant correlations between clients' scores on the MMS and the Weschsler Adult Intelligence Scale (Folstein et al., 1975).

Ordering Information

Available in: Folstein, M.F., Folstein, S.F., & McHugh, P.R. (1975). Mini-Mental State. A practical method for grading the cognitive state of patients for the clinician. *Journal of Psychiatric Research, 12,* 189–198.

STROOP COLOR AND WORD TEST (STROOP)

Purpose

The STROOP (Golden, 1978) was designed to evaluate an individual's ability "to sort information from his or her environment and to selectively react to this information" (Golden, 1978, p. 2).

Description

The STROOP consists of three 8.5 × 11-inch stimulus cards: (1) the words "RED," "BLUE," and "GREEN" are printed in black and white, in random order in 5 columns; (2) the series "XXXX" is printed in 5 columns, with each "XXXX" randomly colored either red, blue, or green; (3) the words "RED," "BLUE," and "GREEN" are printed, in random order in 5 columns, with each word printed in a color different from the color named by the word, e.g "GREEN" might be printed in red or blue. The client's task is to read the color words on the first page, name the colors shown on the second page, and name the color the words are printed in on the third page. Clients get three scores: (1) the Word Score (W) is the number of items completed correctly on the first page, (2) the Color Score (C) is the number of items completed correctly on the second page, and (3) the Color-Word Score (CW) is the number of items completed correctly on the third page.

Method

This is a therapist-administered test that can be given either individually or to groups.

Psychometric Properties

Normative data are available for adults aged 15–80 years, based on six different studies. Test–retest reliability coefficients reported for the three scores are: (1) 0.85–0.89 for the W score, (2) 0.79–0.84 for the C score, and (3) 0.69–0.73 for the CW score. Construct validity is suggested by studies showing children with retardation to have lower STROOP scores than healthy children (Golden, 1978).

Ordering Information

Psychological Assessment Resources (PAR); P.O. Box 998; Odessa, FL 33556; 1-800-331-TEST (8378); FAX: 1-800-727-9329; www.parinc. com

TEST OF EVERYDAY ATTENTION (TEA)

Purpose

The TEA (Robertson, Ward, Ridgeway, & Nimmo-Smith, 1994) was designed to evaluate attention related to everyday activities.

Description

The TEA includes eight subtests: map search, elevator counting, elevator counting with distractions, visual elevator, elevator counting with reversal, telephone search, telephone search while counting, and lottery. The test has three versions that allows testing on successive occasions without practice effect.

Psychometric Properties

In studies with healthy adults taking two versions of the test, test–retest reliability coefficients for the eight subtests ranged from 0.59 to 0.90; coefficients for six of the subtests were above 0.70. Concurrent validity was established through comparisons with other tests of attention. (Zoltan, 1996).

Ordering Information

Psychological Assessment Resources (PAR); P.O. Box 998; Odessa, FL 33556; 1-800-331-TEST (8378); FAX: 1-800-727-9329; www.parinc. com

THE HOOPER VISUAL ORGANIZATION TEST (VOT)

Purpose

The VOT (Hooper, 1985) was designed to measure the ability to organize visual stimuli.

Description

The VOT consists of 30 stimulus items. To create these items, 30 line drawings of simple objects were divided into pieces; the pieces for each object were then arranged in random order within a picture border (Figure D-1). The person taking the test has to visually assemble the object pieces to determine what the objects are, and name the objects. Correct responses are scored as 1 point. The scoring key contains a list of ½ credit responses as well; these are incorrect responses, i.e., perceptual mistakes that are common for healthy adults. A Total Raw Score— the sum of 1 and ½ credit responses—can be converted to a Corrected Raw Score based on the test taker's age and educational level, and to a T score. The test can be administered in less than 15 minutes.

Method

This is a therapist-administered test.

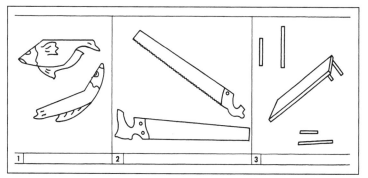

FIGURE D-1. Part of Hooper Visual Organization Test. Selected items for the Hooper Visual Organization Test, copyright © 1957, renewed 1985 by H. Elston Hooper. Reprinted by permission of the publisher, Western Psychological Services, 12031 Wilshire Boulevard, Los Angeles, California, 90025, U.S.A. Not to be reprinted in whole or part for any additional purpose without the expressed, written permission of the publisher. All rights reserved.

Psychometric Properties

Normative T scores are based on a sample of 231 adult males at a VA hospital, age range from 20 to older than 70 years. Split-half reliability has ranged from 0.78 with a sample of 73 incoming clients in a state mental hospital to 0.82, with a sample of healthy college students. Construct and criterion-related validity are supported by several studies that have shown the VOT discriminates between individuals with neurodysfunction and those without neurodysfunction (Western Psychological Services, 1983).

Ordering Information

Western Psychological Services; Publishers and Distributors; 12031 Wilshire Boulevard; Los Angeles, CA 90025-1251; 1-800-648-8857; FAX: (310) 478-2061; www.wpspublish.com

WISCONSIN CARD SORTING TEST (WCST)

Purpose

The WCST (Heaton et al., 1993) was designed to evaluate "abstract reasoning ability and the ability to shift cognitive strategies in response to changing environmental contingencies" (Heaton et al., 1993, p. 1). Clients should have sufficient visual and auditory ability to hear the instructions and visually discriminate between the different colors, shapes, and numbers of shapes illustrated on the test cards.

Description

The WCST consists of four stimulus cards and 128 response cards. The four stimulus cards show: (1) one red triangle, (2) two green stars, (3) three yellow crosses, and (4) four blue circles. These stimulus cards are laid out in front of the client. The client is then given a deck of 64 response cards and asked to match each card from the deck with one of the four stimulus cards. The response cards depict various combinations of the shapes and colors on the stimulus cards, with the number of shapes varying from one to four on any given response card. The response cards could be matched to the stimulus cards according to either color, shape, or number; the therapist keeps one of these sorting principles in mind but does not tell the client which one. The client has to guess the sorting principle by the therapist's indication of whether the matches are correct or incorrect. Once the client has guessed the correct principle and successfully made 10 correct matches using that principle, the therapist changes the sorting principle, indicating this only by telling the client that previously correct matches are now incorrect. Again, once the client has guessed the correct principle and successfully made 10 correct matches using that principle, the therapist changes the sorting principle. Scores are determined by the number of sorts a client needs to guess a sorting principle (establishing set), the client's ability to maintain the sorting principle through 10 trials (maintaining set), and the number of cards the client needs to change the sorting principle (ability to shift set). Matching errors are categorized as perservative (client persists with same sorting principle when given feedback that it is now incorrect) or nonperservative (client is trying different sorting principles to find the new one).

Method

This is a therapist-administered test.

Psychometric Properties

Normative data are available for individuals aged 6.5–89 years; scores corrected for education level are available for adults aged 20 years and older. Normative scores were established with a total sample of 899 healthy subjects. Interrater reliability coefficients have ranged from .88 to .96 for experienced clinicians, and from 0.75 to 0.97 for novice testers. Concurrent validity has been established in two factor analysis studies which showed the WCST loaded on the same factors as other tests of abstract reasoning (Heaton et al., 1993).

Ordering Information

Psychological Assessment Resources (PAR); P.O. Box 998; Odessa, FL 33556; 1-800-331-TEST (8378); FAX: 1-800-727-9329; www.parinc. com

E

MOTOR EVALUATION PROCEDURES

RANGE OF MOTION

General Principles

A neutral zero method for measuring and recording is recommended by the Committee on Joint Motion of the American Academy of Orthopedic Surgeons. Most clinics use this 180 degree system where:

1) 0 degrees is the starting position for all joint motions
2) Anatomic position is the starting position
3) 180 degrees is superimposed as a semi-circle on the body in the plane in which the motion will occur
4) The axis of the joint is the axis of the semi-circle or arc of motion
5) All joint motions begin at 0 degrees and increase toward 180 degrees (Pedretti, 1996a; Trombly, 1995)

Other measurement systems used include the 360 degree system where 180 degrees is a starting position and motion occurs toward 0 degrees (Pedretti, 1996a; Trombly, 1995).

Formal joint measurement is not necessary with every client, especially when limited range of motion is not anticipated. Typical diagnoses that may necessitate closer attention include arthritis, fractures, cerebrovascular accident (CVA), and spinal cord injury. Active range of motion can be visually observed during activities of daily living and/or by having the client move through various positions. All joints can be put briefly through passive range of motion (Pedretti, 1996a).

Normal range of motion varies from one person to the next. Ranges are listed in the literature and on most recording forms. One could also measure the uninvolved extremity as a normal comparison. A medical history should be noted for any previous joint injury or secondary diagnosis affecting range of motion. Range of motion can be limited by pain. Joints should not be forced passed the point of resistance during passive range of motion (Pedretti, 1996a).

When evaluating range of motion, the therapist may need to provide outside support/stability so the individual is free to concentrate and attempt the desired movement as opposed to "fixing" in order to even sit upright. One should also evaluate scapular mobility, thoracic spinal extension, head/neck positioning before proceeding with shoulder joint measurements, as these all affect glenohumeral joint motion (Pedretti, 1996a).

Finally, before actual evaluation, the therapist needs to know average normal range of motion, how the joint moves and how to position him or herself, the client, and the joints for measurement. One should think about comfort as well as body mechanics to protect oneself and the client while placing the goniometer and providing support to the joint being tested.

Range of Motion Evaluation Procedure

1. Position client comfortably.
2. Explain/demonstrate to client what you're doing and why.
3. Stabilize joint proximal to joint being measured.
4. Observe available movement via having client move joint or examiner move joint passively to get a sense of joint mobility.
5. Place goniometer axis over joint axis in starting position. Stationary bar goes over stationary bone proximal to the joint, parallel to the longitudinal axis of the bone. Moveable bar goes over moveable bone distal to the joint, parallel to the longitudinal axis of the bone. Face top of goniometer protractor away from the direction of movement to avoid goniometer dial (end of moveable bar) going off the measurement scale.
6. Record the number of degrees at starting position.
7. Hold the body part securely above and below the joint being measured. Gently move the joint through the available passive range of motion. Do not use excessive force. Note any crepitus. Stop at any point of pain or end or range. The axis of motion for some joints coincides with bony landmarks. Other joint axes are found by observing the movement of the joint to determine the point around which the motion occurs.
8. Return limb to resting position.
9. Record the number of degrees at the final position. Note which position the joint measurement was taken in when more than one position can be used (i.e., shoulder internal/external rotation). Date and sign.

Figures E-1 through E-6 show examples of goniometer measurements. Things that influence accuracy and reliability of goniometer measurement include the type of support given to the body part, bulky clothing, environmental factors such as temperature, time of day, client fatigue, reaction to pain, and examiner experience (LaStays & Wheeler, 1994; Pedretti, 1996a; Riddle, 1992; Wei, McQuade, & Smidt, 1993).

(text continues on page 164)

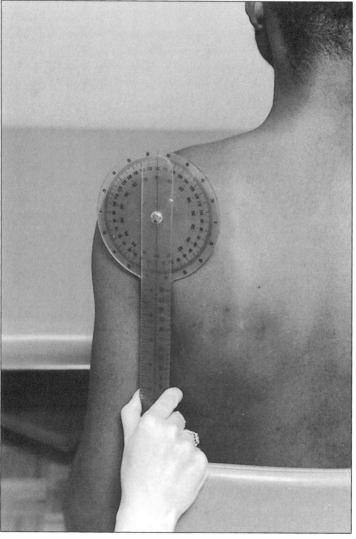

APPENDIX E

FIGURE E-1.   Goniometric Measurement of Shoulder Abduction-starting Position. Photo courtesy of the Rehabilitation Institute of Chicago.

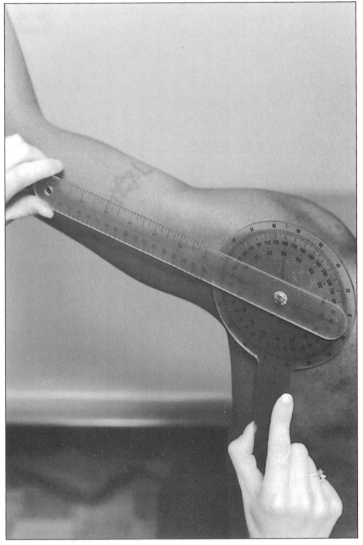

FIGURE E-2. Goniometric Measurement of Shoulder Abduction. Photo courtesy of the Rehabilitation Institute of Chicago.

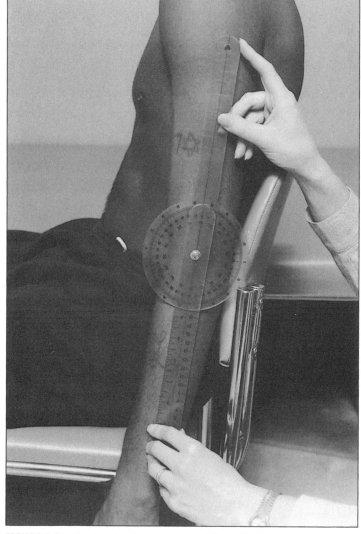

FIGURE E-3.   Goniometric Measurement of Elbow Flexion-starting Position.
Photo courtesy of the Rehabilitation Institute of Chicago.

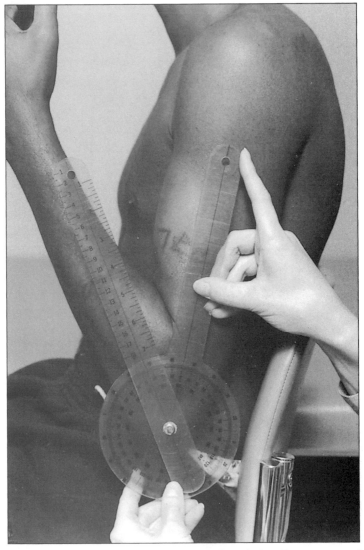

FIGURE E-4.   Goniometric Measurement of Elbow Flexion. Photo courtesy of the Rehabilitation Institute of Chicago.

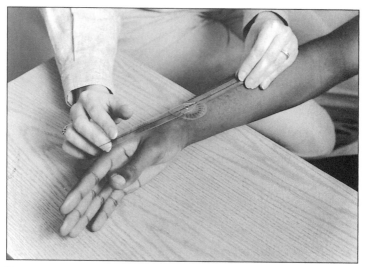

FIGURE E-5. Goniometric Measurement of Wrist Extension-starting Position. Photo courtesy of the Rehabilitation Institute of Chicago.

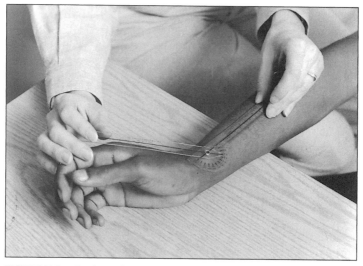

FIGURE E-6. Goniometric Measurement of Wrist Extension. Photo courtesy of the Rehabilitation Institute of Chicago.

Recording Results

When using the 180 degree system, the evaluator should record the number of degrees at the starting position and the number of degrees at the final position after the joint has passed through the maximal possible arc of motion. Normal range of motion starts at 0 degrees and increases toward 180 degrees. A limitation can be indicated at either end of the scale; For example:

elbow	0–140 degrees	normal
	20–140 degrees	limited extension
	0–100 degrees	limited flexion

(Pedretti, 1996a)
Figure E-7 and Figure 2-29 show sample forms for recording range of motion measurements.

Interpreting Results

A therapist should focus on ranges that fall below functional limits, that is, the amount of joint range necessary to perform activities of daily living without the use of special equipment. Evaluate what is causing the decreased range. Is it pain, edema, muscle weakness, skin

FIGURE E-7.   Form for Recording Upper Extremity Range of Motion, Strength, and Edema From Cedars-Sinai Upper Extremity Initial Evaluation Profile. Reprinted with permission of Cedars-Sinai Medical Center.

adhesions, spasticity, bony obstruction or destruction, or soft tissue contracture? Is the cause changeable? Can you increase active range or prevent further loss via stretching, strengthening, orthotic management, casting, or modalities? Treatment goals should reflect the identified problem. If the available range is not expected to change, one should focus on adaptive techniques and/or use of adaptive equipment to perform the desired task (Pedretti, 1996a; Trombly, 1995).

MUSCLE TONE

Methods of Measurement

To date, it has been difficult to achieve both reliability and validity when measuring muscle tone. There is no standardized procedure. Various electromyographic, biomechanical, and myotonometric methods have varying degrees of success. Often, evaluation equipment is expensive and more suited to research than clinical applications (Undzis et al, 1996; Worley et al, 1991).

Clinically, numerous methods exist. The most common method of measuring tone is via grasping the body part gently, firmly and moving it briskly through the desired movement pattern. The Ashworth (1964) scale grades tone from a 0 (no increase in tone) to a 4 (limb is rigid in flexion or extension). Bohannan and Smith (1987) modified Ashworth's scale by adding an additional level, incorporating the angle at which resistance appeared, and controlling the speed of passive movement with a one-second count (Table E-1).

Brennan (1959) measured range of motion that is possible before resistance to movement is felt. King (1987) established a five-point rating scale for each of four functions: presence of tone, active range of motion, alternating movement, and resistance to passive movement. Bobath (1978) described a method of evaluating the combined effects of tone and primitive reflexes. Clients limbs are moved in normal patterns of usage and the adaptation of the different muscle groups to changes in position are noted. Fugl-Meyer, Jaasko, Leyman, Olson, and Steglind (1975) established an objective method to measure function as well as movement in hemiparetic clients (Table E-2).

Recording Results

When recording results, one should note the position in which testing was done, the presence of abnormal reflexes, as well as any external factors that may influence results. This may include environmental

TABLE E-1	MODIFIED ASHWORTH SCALE

Grade	Description
0	No increase in muscle tone
1	Slight increase in tone, manifested by a catch and release or by minimal resistance at the end of the range of motion (ROM) when the affected part(s) is moved in flexion or extension
+1	Slight increase in muscle tone, manifested by a catch, followed by minimal resistance throughout the remainder (less than half) of the ROM
2	More marked increase in muscle tone through most of the ROM, but affected parts(s) easily moved
3	Considerable increase in muscle tone, passive movement difficult
4	Affected part(s) rigid in flexion or extension

Reprinted from Bohannon, R.W. & Smith, R.B., "Interrater reliability of a modified Ashworth Scale of muscle spasticity," *Physical Therapy,* 1987, 67, p. 207, with permission of the American Physical Therapy Association

TABLE E-2	FUGL-MEYER SCALE OF FUNCTIONAL RETURN AFTER HEMIPLEGIA

Grade	Movement of the shoulder, elbow, forearm, and lower extremity
I	Muscle stretch reflexes can be elicited
II	Volitional movements can be performed within the dynamic flexor/extensor synergies
III	Volitional motion is performed mixing dynamic flexor and extensor synergies
IV	Volitional movements are performed with little or no synergy dependence
V	Normal muscle stretch reflexes

Reprinted with permission from Kohlmeyer, K. (1998), Evaluation of sensory and neuromuscular performance components. In M.E. Neistadt & E.B. Crepeau (Eds.), *Willard & Spackman's occupational therapy* (9th ed.) (pp. 223–260). Philadelphia: Lippincott, p. 236.

temperature, time of day, and medications. One should note the presence, degree, distribution, and type of abnormal tone as well as its impact on the client's ability to perform activities of daily living. This can be done graphically, with a table, and/or in narrative form.

Interpreting Results

If a client has abnormal tone, one should ask several questions. First of all, does it affect function? What influences the tone—position of the head, hips, or trunk? Does a combination of muscle tone exist? Do medications have a pharmacological effect? Do facilitation and/or inhibitory techniques have any short-term or long-term effect?

If low tone is present, a muscle test can determine the degree of weakness. If recovery from low tone is expected, graded exercise and therapeutic activity is appropriate. Adaptive equipment may be necessary on a short-term or long-term basis. Positioning should protect weak muscles from overstretching.

High muscle tone necessitates techniques to maintain range of motion, perform activities of daily living and positioning in patterns opposite to spastic patterns. Inhibitory techniques depend on the nature and severity of the disability, abnormal tone distribution, and other concomitant problems (Undzis et al., 1996; Warren, 1991; Mathiowetz & Haugen, 1995).

MUSCLE STRENGTH

General Principles

Gross muscle testing evaluates the strength of groups of muscles that perform specific movements at each joint (i.e., elbow flexors). Manual muscle testing evaluates individual muscles (i.e., biceps, brachialis, brachioradialis). A therapist might first observe functional performance and then decide to focus on a certain muscle group based on the outcome of the observation. Certain diagnoses such as spinal cord injury, Guillan Barré, and peripheral nerve injury may necessitate specific muscle testing as opposed to a diagnosis of generalized weakness, lower extremity amputee or hip replacement, which lend themselves to gross muscle testing.

To perform muscle testing, a therapist needs to know muscles and their functions, anatomical position and direction of muscle fibers, and angle of pull on joints. Substitution patterns (i.e., when a muscle or muscle group attempts to compensate for lack of function in a weak or paralyzed muscle) should be expected and targeted (i.e., shoulder

APPENDIX E

external rotation and eccentric lengthening of biceps versus triceps elbow extension in gravity eliminated position).

Muscle testing cannot be used accurately with clients who have upper motor neuron disorders. In these clients, hypertonicity muscle tone and movement tend to occur in gross synergistic patterns and may be influenced by primitive reflexes (Pedretti, 1996b). Note that in spinal cord injury, which is an upper motor neuron disorder, the muscles being tested are those innervated by spinal cord segments above the level of the injury.

Gravity influences muscle function. Gravity-eliminated positions are used with (O-P+/0–2+) grades. Movements against gravity are used with (F-N/3–5) grades. Definitions for muscle grades are relatively standard (see Table 2-20).

Assignment of muscle grades depend on clinical judgment, knowledge and examiner experience. The amount of resistance given (i.e., slight, moderate, or full) is determined by the client's age, sex, body type, and occupation. The amount of resistance given also varies from one muscle group to the next. One must consider the size and relative muscle power and leverage used when giving resistance. That is, one wouldn't apply the same force to finger flexors as to shoulder flexors (Daniels & Worthingham, 1986; Kendall, McCreary, & Provance, 1993; Pedretti, 1996b; Rancho, 1978; Trombly, 1995a).

In individual cases, positioning for muscle testing in the correct plane may not be possible due to medical precautions, immobilization devices, trunk instability, or weakness. Modifications in positioning and grading are cited for individual tests in muscle testing manuals (Daniels & Worthingham, 1986; Kendall et al., 1993). Lamb (1985) discusses various aspects of manual muscle testing including variables of testing procedures, reliability, and validity issues. Differences in methodology (i.e., force application, stabilization, and positioning) and strength determination during controlled studies are discussed by Smidt and Roger (1982).

Procedure for Muscle Testing

Whether performing gross or manual muscle testing, certain general procedures apply:

1) Determine available passive range of motion of the joint of muscles being examined.
2) Position and stabilize the body part proximal to part being tested.
3) Demonstrate/describe test motion.
4) Ask client to perform movement.

5) Palpate via placing fingerpads firmly and gently over muscle tendon or belly.
6) Observe client's movement.
7) Ask client to hold position.
8) For grades above Fair/3, resist
   a) in the opposite direction of test movement,
   b) at the end of available range of motion,
   c) on the distal end of the moving bone,
   d) as close to a perpendicular direction as possible (Pedretti, 1996b).

Box E-1 suggests a sequence of muscle testing that streamlines the clinical evaluation process. Figures E-8 through E-13 illustrate specific muscle testing techniques in both gravity eliminated and against gravity po-

---

BOX E-1	SUGGESTED SEQUENCE FOR MUSCLE TESTING

BACKLYING (SUPINE)
Grades N to F
Scapula abduction and upward rotation
Shoulder horizontal abduction
All tests for forearm, wrist, and fingers can be given in the backlying position if necessary

Grades P to O
Shoulder abduction
Elbow flexion
Elbow extension
Hip abduction
Hip adduction
Hip external rotation
Hip internal rotation
Foot inversion
Foot eversion

FACELYING (PRONE)
Grades N to F
Scapula depression
Scapula adduction
Scapula adduction and downward rotation
Shoulder extension
Shoulder external rotation
Shoulder internal rotation
Shoulder horizontal abduction
Elbow extension
Hip extension
Knee flexion
Ankle plantar flexion

continued

APPENDIX E

BOX E-1	SUGGESTED SEQUENCE FOR MUSCLE TESTING (CONTINUED)

Grades P to O
Scapula elevation
Scapula depression
Scapula adduction
Sidelying
Grades N to F
Hip abduction
Hip adduction
Foot inversion
Foot eversion

Grades P to O
Shoulder flexion
Shoulder extension
Hip flexion
Hip extension
Knee flexion
Knee extension
Ankle plantar flexion
Ankle dorsiflexion

SITTING
Grades N to F
Scapula elevation
Shoulder flexion
Shoulder abduction
Elbow flexion
All forearm, wrist, finger, and thumb movements
Hip flexion
Hip external rotation
Hip internal rotation
Knee extension
Ankle dorsiflexion with inversion

Grades P to O
All forearm, wrist, finger, and thumb movements
Ankle dorsiflexion with inversion

Reprinted with permission from Pedretti, L.W. (1996). Evaluation of muscle strength. In L.W. Pedretti (Ed.). *Occupational therapy: Practice skills for physical dysfunction* (4th ed) (p. 117). St. Louis: C.V. Mosby Co.

sitions for: (a) shoulder abduction (middle deltoid), (b) elbow flexion (biceps), and (c) wrist extension (extensor carpi radialis longus).

Hand Strength

For evaluation of hand strength, the American Society of Hand Therapists (ASHT) recommends standard methods of measurement on

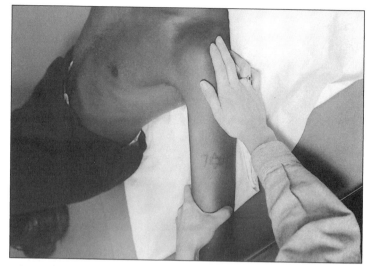

FIGURE E-8.   Muscle Testing for Shoulder Abduction (Middle Deltoid) in Gravity-eliminated Position. Photo courtesy of the Rehabilitation Institute of Chicago.

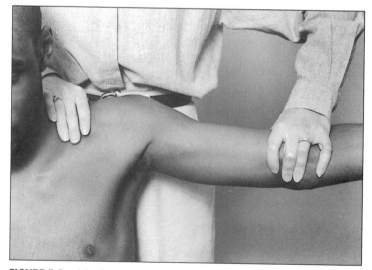

FIGURE E-9.   Muscle Testing for Shoulder Abduction (Middle Deltoid) in Against-gravity position. Photo courtesy of the Rehabilitation Institute of Chicago.

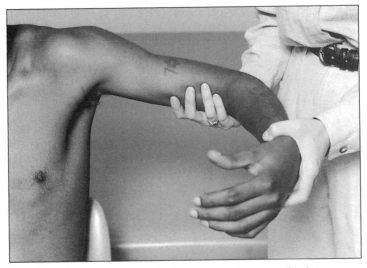

FIGURE E-10. Muscle Testing for Elbow Flexion (Biceps) in Gravity-eliminated Position. Photo courtesy of the Rehabilitation Institute of Chicago.

which norms are based. Standardized positioning and instructions are also recommended by Mathiowetz, Volland, Kashman, and Weber (1984). Grip strength is measured by a standard adjustable handle dynamometer. The subject is seated, shoulder adducted, elbow flexed at 90 degrees and forearm in neutral position. An average of three successive forceful grips is taken (Figure E-14) (Pedretti, 1996b; Trombly 1995, Smith, 1993).

Pinch strength is tested on a standard pinch dynamometer in three ways:

1) TIP pinch—thumb tip to index finger
2) Lateral pinch—thumb pulp to lateral aspect of middle phalanx of index finger
3) Three-point pinch—thumb tip to tips of index and long fingers

An average of three successive trials is taken (Pedretti, 1996b; Smith 1993; Trombly, 1995). See Figures E-15 and E-16 for illustrations of a pinch dynamometer.

Swelling in the hand can affect joint mobility and muscle strength. Swelling can be measured with a volumeter or with circumferential measurements taken with a tape measure. The volumeter measures the amount of water displaced by the hand and is useful for measuring generalized edema (Figure E-17). The uninvolved hand can be

(text continues on page 177)

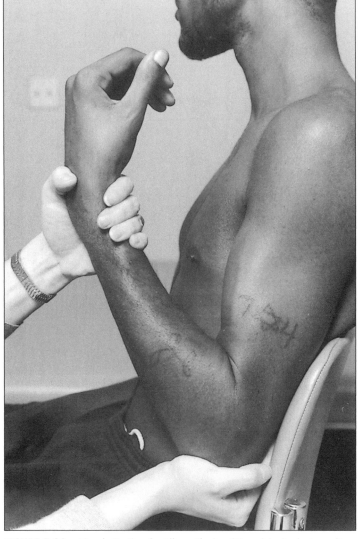

FIGURE E-11.   Muscle Testing for Elbow Flexion (Biceps) in Against-gravity Position. Photo courtesy of the Rehabilitation Institute of Chicago.

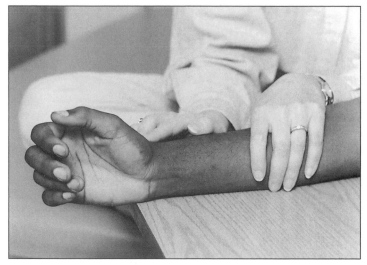

FIGURE E-12. Muscle Testing for Wrist Extension (Extensor Carpi Radialis Longus) in Gravity-eliminated Position. Photo courtesy of the Rehabilitation Institute of Chicago.

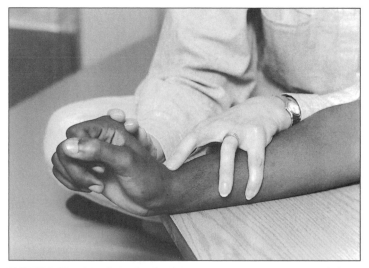

FIGURE E-13. Muscle Testing for Wrist Extension (Extensor Carpi Radialis Longus) in Against-gravity Position. Photo courtesy of the Rehabilitation Institute of Chicago.

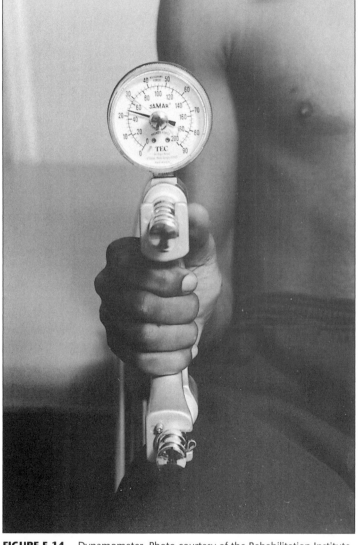

FIGURE E-14.   Dynamometer. Photo courtesy of the Rehabilitation Institute of Chicago.

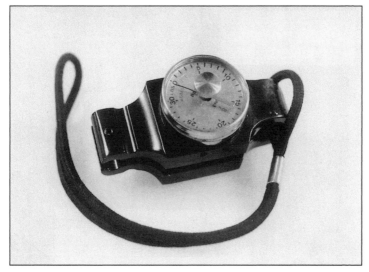

FIGURE E-15.   Pinch Meter. Photo courtesy of the Rehabilitation Institute of Chicago.

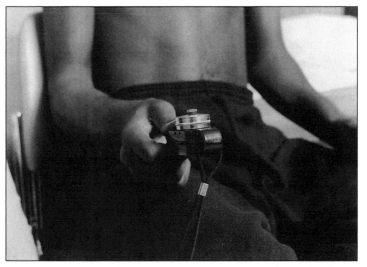

FIGURE E-16.   Pinch Meter Measurement of Lateral Pinch. Photo courtesy of the Rehabilitation Institute of Chicago.

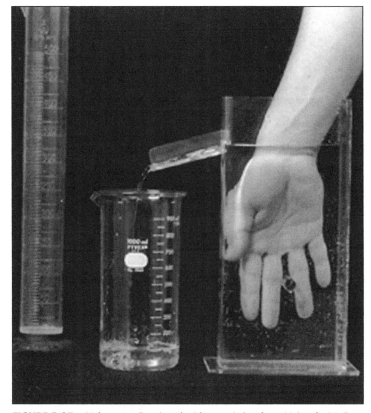

FIGURE E-17. Volumeter. Reprinted with permission from Neistadt, M. E., & Crepeau, E. B. (Eds.), *Willard & Spackman's occupational therapy* (*9th ed., p. 250*). Philadelphia, PA: Lippincott.

measured as a normal comparison. For clients with open wounds or infections, the volumeter may be contraindicated (Fess, 1993). Circumferential measurements are useful for more localized edema, e.g., around a specific joint (Figure E-18). Figure E-7 shows a form for recording circumferential measurements for edema.

Oral Motor Control

Some occupational therapists evaluate and treat oral motor control problems. This can be done alone or in conjunction with a speech and language pathologist. In some work settings occupational therapists do not address this area at all.

Dysphagia is defined as difficulty in swallowing. Swallowing is a

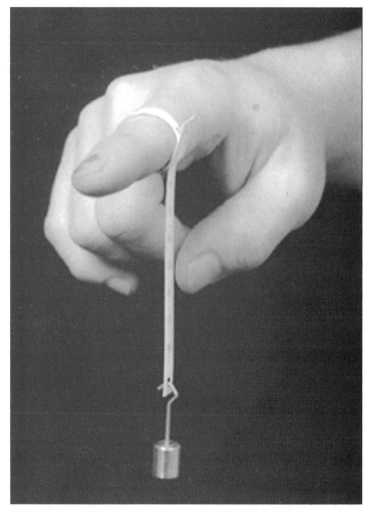

FIGURE E-18.   Circumferential Measurement of Edema With a Tape
Measure. Reprinted with permission from Neistadt, M. E., & Crepeau, E. B.
(Eds.), *Willard & Spackman's occupational therapy* (9th ed., p. 250). *Philadelphia,
PA: Lippincott.*

multistage sequence that, when normally elicited, momentarily blocks
the opening to the respiratory tract as food or beverage is passed
through the pharynx, and into the esophagus. Swallowing can occur
either by willful cortical initiation or by a reflex elicited independently
from higher brain centers (Miller, Groher, Yorkston & Rees, 1988).

Swallowing has three phases: (a) oral—preparation of the bolus or
mass of chewed food; (b) pharyngeal—bolus is propelled through the

pharynx away from the airway, and (c) esophageal—a primary peristaltic wave that propels the bolus through the lower esophageal sphincter and into the stomach.

When dysphagia is recognized or a swallowing complaint registered, the examination should include the following: (a) a complete medical history, (b) a description of the complaint and associated symptoms, (c) a physical examination of the peripheral deglutitive motor and sensory system, and (d) motion radiographic studies (Miller et al., 1988).

Nasal regurgitation is a symptom associated with weakness of the palatopharyngeal mechanism. Aspiration of food or liquid into the "windpipe" is a common complaint of clients with neurological impairment of the swallowing muscles. In the case of dysphagia for solids, a feeling of blockage is common:

Occupational therapy examination includes evaluation of:

1) mental status
2) strength of muscles of the face, mouth, neck, and trunk
3) oral sensation
4) primitive reflexes
5) intraoral mucosa
6) the adequacy of swallowing
(Miller et al., 1988; Nelson, 1996)

APPENDIX E

Recording Results

Figures E-7 and 2-29 show sample forms for recording results of muscle strength testing. The timing of re-evaluation may be dependent on the expected recovery rate, length of stay in therapy, and department protocol. Keep in mind, the focus of therapy, should be an increase in function, not necessarily an increase in the component area of strength.

Interpreting Results

Performing a muscle test is only one component of evaluation. How a therapist interprets and utilizes the information is more important. Some considerations are as follows:

1) Is the problem one of strength, endurance, or a combination? Endurance is the number of repetitions of muscle contraction before fatigue. If endurance is the issue, the therapist needs to emphasize repetitive movements (at less than maximal contraction) to increase endurance.

2) Is the result of your evaluation influenced by impaired tactile sensation and/or proprioception?
3) What is the diagnosis or expected course of the disease? Is there an expected recovery period? Progression of decline? Periods of exacerbation or remission?
4) The degree of weakness, distribution and pattern of weakness (i.e., generalized or specific), and muscle imbalance between agonists and antagonists suggest the type of intervention (i.e., resistive exercises, active assistive activities, orthotic intervention).
5) Coordinate the therapy program with other professionals so that timing/type of appointments and goals are in line with other interventions (Pedretti, 1996b).

REFLEX TESTING

The following principles should be noted when testing primitive reflexes:

1) Reflexes and responses should be tested in several developmental postures.
2) Any stress can release elements of primitive postural reflexes in both the neurologically intact as well as neurologically impaired population.
3) Clients with chronic neuromotor pathology will rarely demonstrate a primitive postural reflex in its pure form. Most often, reflexes are combined so that clients demonstrate elements of several reflexes in one behavioral response (Farber, 1991a,b).
4) Reflexes are usually tested in developmental sequence.

Tables E-3 through E-8 give an overview of various levels of reflex testing.

Innate Primary Reactions

Innate primary reactions are primitive reflexes found in newborns that involve total patterns of flexion and extension (Table E-3).

Automatic Movement Reflexes

Automatic movement reactions are produced by changes of the position of the head in space (Table E-4).

TABLE E-3 | INNATE PRIMARY REACTIONS

Reflex/Reaction	Reflex/Reaction Age Range	Test Position	Stimulus	Response
REFLEX STEPPING	Birth–3 months	Supported in upright position with some weight bearing on feet	Lean client forward; pressure of feet on supporting surface	Rhythmic alternating stepping
GRASP REFLEX	Birth–3 to 4 months	Any—usually supine	Pressure in palm of hand or ulnar side	Flexing of fingers, grasping of stimulus object
PLACING REACTION	Birth–2 months	Sitting or Supine	Brush dorsum of one of the client's hands again the under edge of a table or edge of a stiff cardboard	Flexion of the arm with placement of the hand on to the tabletop
SUCKING REFLEX	Birth–2 months	Any	Stimulation to lips, gums or front of tongue	Sucking, swallowing motions
ROOTING REFLEX	Birth–4 months	Any	Touch/Stroke outward on corner of lips or on cheek	Lower lip, tongue and head more toward stimulus

(Mathiowetz & Haugen, 1995: Simon & Daub, 1993; Sroufe, Cooper, & Deltart, 1992)
Reprinted with permission from Kohlmeyer, K. (1998), Evaluation of sensory and neuromuscular performance components. In M.E. Neistadt & E.B. Crepeau (Eds.), *Willard & Spackman's occupational therapy* (9th ed.) (pp. 223–260). Philadelphia: Lippincott, p. 251.

APPENDIX E

TABLE E-4 | AUTOMATIC MOVEMENT REFLEXES

Reflex	Reflex Age Range	Test Position	Stimulus	Response
MORO REFLEX	Birth–5 months	Semi-reclining or supine	Dropping head backward from a semi-sitting position or a loud noise near the head	Extension or flexion and abduction of arms and spreading of fingers
LANDAU REFLEX	4 months–12 to 24 months	Prone, suspended in space with support under the chest	Passive or Active neck extension	Back and legs extend
PROTECTIVE EXTENSOR THRUST	6 months–remainder of life	Sitting or Prone	Displace body forward, side-ways and backwards (separately)	Protective extension of limb to protect head

(Mathiowetz & Haugen, 1995: Simon & Daub, 1993; Sroufe, Cooper, & Deltart, 1992)
Reprinted with permission from Kohlmeyer, K. (1998), Evaluation of sensory and neuromuscular performance components. In M.E. Neistadt & E.B. Crepeau (Eds.), *Willard & Spackman's occupational therapy* (9th ed.) (pp. 223–260). Philadelphia: Lippincott, p. 251.

Spinal Level Reflexes

Reflexes mediated at the spinal level are phasic in nature and are basic to mobility motor patterns (Table E-5).

Brainstem Level Reflexes

Reflexes mediated at the brain stem level are static, postural reflexes that cause a change in muscle tone throughout the body. The changed tone is in response to a change of the position of the head in space or in relation to the body which activates the vestibular system; the changed tone is maintained as long as the stimulus is present (Table E-6).

Midbrain Level Reactions

A reaction is a stereotyped, non-obligatory response to a particular stimulus. Midbrain reactions permit the development of maturationally acquired motor milestones. Righting reactions are integrated at this level and interact with one another to effect the normal head-to-body relationship in space and to each other (Table E-7).

Cortical Reactions

Cortical level reactions are the result of the efficient interaction of the cerebral cortex, basal ganglia, and the cerebellum. Equilibrium reactions occur when muscle tone is normalized and enable the adaptation to changes in the body's center of gravity. They are the integration of vestibular, visual, and tactile inputs (Table E-8).

Recording Results

Test position(s) should be noted. Results are usually recorded as to whether the client's response is positive or negative. Intensity (i.e., the speed of response and degree of change) as well as quality (i.e., which components of the response are present under which conditions) of responses should be documented. Figure 2-27 shows a sample form for recording equilibrium reactions.

Interpreting Results

Obligatory reflexive responses such as domination of a postural reflex indicates severe central nervous system pathology. Disturbance of higher integrating centers manifests in evidence of a reflex but not

(text continues on page 189)

APPENDIX E

TABLE E-5 | SPINAL LEVEL REFLEXES

Reflex	Reflex Age Range	Test Position	Stimulus	Response
FLEXOR WITHDRAWAL	Birth–2 months	Supine or sitting with head in midposition, legs extended	Stimulation to sole of foot	Uncontrolled flexion of stimulated leg
EXTENSOR THRUST	Birth–2 months	Supine or sitting with head in midposition. One leg is in extension and the other leg is fully flexed	Pressure to the ball of the foot of the flexed leg	Uncontrolled extension of the stimulated leg
CROSSED EXTENSION	Birth–2 months	Supine with head in midposition. One leg is in extension and the other leg is fully flexed	Passively flex the extended leg	Extension of the opposite leg with hip internal rotation and adduction

(Mathiowetz & Haugen, 1995: Simon & Daub, 1993; Sroufe, Cooper, & Deltart, 1992)
Reprinted with permission from Kohlmeyer, K. (1998). Evaluation of sensory and neuromuscular performance components. In M.E. Neistadt & E.B. Crepeau (Eds.), *Willard & Spackman's occupational therapy* (9th ed.) (pp. 223–260). Philadelphia: Lippincott, p. 252.

TABLE E-6 | BRAINSTEM REFLEXES

Reflex	Reflex Age Range	Test Position	Stimulus	Response
ASYMMETRICAL TONIC NECK REFLEX (ATNR)	Birth–4 to 6 months	Supine or Sitting with arms and legs extended. Clients with minimal reflexes responses can be tested in quadruped.	Passively or Actively turn the head 90 degrees to one side.	Increase of extensor tone of limbs on the face side and flexor tone of limbs on the skull side
SYMMETRICAL TONIC NECK REFLEX (STNR)	Birth–4 to 6 months	Sitting or Quadruped	1. Flex client's head and bring chin toward chest 2. Extend client's head	1. Flexion of upper extremities and extension of lower extremities 2. Extension of upper extremities and flexion of lower extremities
TONIC LABYRINTHINE REFLEX (TLR)	Birth–4 months	Prone with head in midposition	Test position is the stimulus	Flexion of the extremities or increase in flexor tone
TONIC LABYRINTHINE REFLEX-SUPINE	Birth–4 months	Supine with head in midposition	Test position is the stimulus	Extension of the extremities or increase in extensor tone

continued

| TABLE E-6 | BRAINSTEM REFLEXES (CONTINUED) |

Reflex	Reflex Age Range	Test Position	Stimulus	Response
POSITIVE SUPPORTING REACTION	Birth–6 months	Standing, Supine or Sitting	Firmly contact the ball of the foot to the floor; or footboard of the bed and dorsiflex the foot	Rigid extension of lower extremity due to cocontraction of flexors and extensors of knee and hip joints
ASSOCIATED REACTIONS	Associated movements are normal throughout life when attempting strenuous activities. Associated reactions are stereotyped tonic reactions by which one extremity influences the posture of another extremity.	Any position	Resist any motion or have client squeeze an object with unaffected hand.	The motion used as a stimulus will be mimicked by the other hand.

(Mathiowetz & Haugen, 1995: Simon & Daub, 1993; Sroufe, Cooper, & Deltart, 1992) Reprinted with permission from Kohlmeyer, K. (1998), Evaluation of sensory and neuromuscular performance components. In M.E. Neistadt & E.B. Crepeau (Eds.), *Willard & Spackman's occupational therapy* (9th ed.) (pp. 223–260). Philadelphia: Lippincott, p. 252.

TABLE E-7 | MIDBRAIN REACTIONS

Reaction	Reaction Age Range	Test Position	Stimulus	Response
NECK RIGHTING	Birth–6 months	Supine w/arms and legs extended	Passively turn head to one side and hold it there	Body rotates as a whole in the direction to which the head was turned
LABYRINTHINE RIGHTING ACTING ON THE HEAD	2 months–throughout life	Prone supine or vertical positions in space. Subject's vision is occluded	Prone or supine positions are test stimuli or in vertical position body is tilted laterally	Head seeks vertical position in space
BODY RIGHTING ACTING ON THE HEAD	6 months–5 years	Client is blindfolded 1. Prone 2. Supine	Asymmetric stimulation of the pressure sense organs on the anterior of the body surface	Head is brought into a face vertical position that orients it to the surface with which client is in contact
BODY RIGHTING ON THE BODY	6 months–18 months	Supine with arms and legs extended	Passively or actively turn the head to one side	Segmental rotation around the body axis toward the direction of the head

Mathiowetz & Haugen, 1995: Simon & Daub, 1993; Sroufe, Cooper, & Deltart, 1992; Trombly & Scott, 1989)
Reprinted with permission from Kohlmeyer, K. (1998), Evaluation of sensory and neuromuscular performance components. In M.E. Neistadt & E.B. Crepeau (Eds.), *Willard & Spackman's occupational therapy* (9th ed.) (pp. 223–260). Philadelphia: Lippincott, p. 253.

TABLE E-8 | CORTICAL REACTIONS

Reaction	Reaction Age Range	Test Position	Stimulus	Response
OPTIC RIGHTING	2 months–throughout life	Prone or Supine on a raised mat sitting with the head laterally flexed. Eyes are open	Position of the head in relation to landmarks in space	Head is raised upright in space
EQUILIBRIUM REACTION	Depends on test position —throughout life	Supine (7–8 months) Prone (5 months) Quadruped (9–12 months) Sitting (6 months) Kneel—Standing (15 months) Standing (15 months)	Rocking client or supporting surface sufficiently to disturb balance	Automatic movements to maintain balance, right head and body; protective reactions

(Mathiowetz & Haugen, 1995: Simon & Daub, 1993; Sroufe, Cooper, & Deltart, 1992; Trombly & Scott, 1989)
Reprinted with permission from Kohlmeyer, K. (1998). Evaluation of sensory and neuromuscular performance components. In M.E. Neistadt & E.B. Crepeau (Eds.), Willard & Spackman's occupational therapy (9th ed.) (pp. 223–260). Philadelphia: Lippincott, p. 254.

188

complete domination (Farber, 1991a,b). For example, a weak reflex response would be tonal changes in the extremities as opposed to actual movement. This should not be confused with tonal changes in a stimulus neutral condition. Problems with reflex integration result in decreased: (a) trunk segmentation, (b) ability to perform isolated movement, (c) adaptation of muscles to postural change, (d) function of anti-gravity muscles, and increased synergistic movement. Formal assessment should always be accompanied by observing how reflexes effect motor and functional performance. For example, a positive asymmetrical tonic neck reflex (ATNR) can prevent rolling from supine to prone due to scapular retraction on the skull side extremity (which prevents bringing that arm across) and an extended arm on the face side (Trombly & Scott, 1989).

ENDURANCE

Endurance can be defined as the ability to sustain a given activity over time. It is related to cardiopulmonary, biomechanical, and neuromuscular function (Asmussen, 1979; Farber, 1991a,b; Lunsford, 1978; Trombly, 1995a). Endurance is a measure of stamina and fitness which can be compromised by inactivity, immobilization, cardiorespiratory deconditioning, muscular deconditioning, and diminished flexibility.

Endurance is related to intensity, duration, and frequency of activity. It can be reported as a percentage of maximal heart rate, a number of repetitions over time, or the amount of time a contraction can be held (Trombly, 1995).

Cardiorespiratory Endurance

Cardiorespiratory endurance is defined by the American College of Sports Medicine (1991) as "the ability to perform large-muscle, dynamic, moderate-to-high intensity exercises for prolonged periods" (p. 39). Cardiorespiratory endurance depends on the functional states of the respiratory, cardiovascular, and musculoskeletal systems. Maximal oxygen uptake (abbreviated VO_2 max) is a standard measure of cardiorespiratory endurance. VO_2 max is a measure of the maximal amount of oxygen that a person can take in and dispense during exercise and is related to a person's maximal metabolic equivalent (MET) capacity (American College of Sports Medicine, 1991). "One MET is equivalent to an oxygen uptake of 3.5 [milliliters per kilogram body weight per minute]. It is conventional in exercise testing to express VO_2 max in METS (e.g., VO_2 max of 35 [milliliters per kilogram body weight per minute] is equivalent to 10 METS)" (American College of Sports Medicine, 1991, p. 16). VO_2 max measurements require sophisticated equipment; occupational therapists are not qualified to make these measurements but can use other indicators of cardiorespiratory endurance related to VO_2 max—MET levels of activity and heart rate responses to activity.

To measure MET levels of activities, an occupational therapist can consult a MET table that indicates the average number of METS expended for given activities (Table E-9). These tables report MET levels that have been established by exercise physiology research; the MET level values reported represent the average number of the METS expended by a 150-pound person. Heavier people will expend more METS and lighter people will expend fewer METS than the values indicated on a MET table for any given activity. Additionally, MET levels vary with stress and environmental conditions (American College of Sports Medicine, 1991). Therefore, a MET table represents only an APPROXIMATE range of MET expenditure for any given activity and should be reported as such. For example, an OTS could report that a client who was able to get dressed without experiencing shortness of breath or an increase in heart rate of more than 20 beats per minute could tolerate activities of approximately 2.5–3.5 METS (Trombly, 1989).

Clients' specific heart rate responses to activity need to be recorded in addition to MET levels. Heart rate quantifies the physiological demand of an activity; in healthy individuals higher heart rates correspond to higher oxygen consumption. This is not true for persons with cardiopulmonary diseases because these diseases disrupt normal physiological responses to activity. Heart rate responses to treatment activities can be related to a person's maximal heart rate as a percentage of maximum. For persons without cardiopulmonary disease, maximum heart rate can be determined by the formula: 220 − age. In persons with cardiopulmonary disease, maximum heart rate should be determined by an exercise stress test administered by a cardiologist (American College of Sports Medicine, 1991).

Biomechanical/Neuromuscular Endurance

Biomechanical neuromuscular endurance refers to the capacity of a muscle or muscle group to sustain a contraction over time. In normal muscle, only a few of available motor units are needed at any one time as active and resting units take turns. "However, if a person sustains a contraction that exceeds 15 to 20% maximum voluntary contraction (MVC) for the muscle group involved, blood flow to the working

TABLE E-9	METABOLIC EQUIVALENT (MET) VALUES FOR SOME OCCUPATIONAL PERFORMANCE AREAS

MET LEVELS (Oxygen consumed) [Level of Activity]	SELF-CARE ACTIVITIES	WORK AND PRODUCTIVE ACTIVITIES	PLAY AND LEISURE ACTIVITIES
1.5–2.0 METS (4–7 ml/kg/min) [Very light/Minimal]	Eating Shaving, grooming Getting in and out of bed Standing Walking (1.6 km or 1 mph)	Desk work Typing Writing	Playing cards Sewing Knitting
2–3 METS (7–11 ml/kg/min) [Light]	Showering in warm water Level walking (3.25 km or 2 mph)	Ironing Light wood-working Riding lawn mower	Level bicycling (8 km or 5 mph) Billiards Bowling Golfing with power cart
3–4 METS (11–14 ml/kg/min) [Moderate]	Dressing, undressing Walking (5 km or 3 mph)	Cleaning windows Making beds Mopping floors Vacuuming Bricklaying Machine assembly	Bicycling (10 km or 6 mph) Fly fishing (standing in waders) Horseshoe pitching
4–5 METS (14–18 ml/kg/min) [Heavy]	Showering in hot water Walking (5.5 km or 3.5 mph)	Scrubbing floors Hoeing Raking leaves Light carpentry	Bicycling (13 km or 8 mph) Table tennis Tennis (doubles)
5–6 METS (18–21 ml/kg/min) [Heavy]	Walking (6.5 km or 4 mph)	Digging in garden Shoveling light earth	Bicycling (16 km or 10 mph) Canoeing (6.5 km or 4 mph) Ice or roller skating (15 km or 9 mph)
6–7 METS (21–25 ml/kg/min) [Very Heavy]	Walking (8 km or 5 mph)	Snow shoveling Splitting wood	Bicycling (17.5 km or 11 mph) Light downhill skiing Ski touring (4 km or 2.5 mph)

Note. ml/kg/min = milliliters of oxygen consumed per kilogram body weight per minute; km = kilometer; mph = miles per hour
(Atchison, 1995; Brannon, Foley, Starr, & Black, 1993; Trombly, 1989). Reprinted with permission from Kohlmeyer, K. (1998). Evaluation of sensory and neuromuscular performance components. In M. E. Neistadt & E. B. Crepeau (Eds.), *Willard & Spackman's occupational therapy* (9th ed.) (pp. 223– 260). Philadelphia: Lippincott, p. 255.

APPENDIX E

muscles will decrease, causing a shift to anaerobic metabolism which limits duration (Dehn, 1980)" (Trombly, 1995, p. 153). Anaerobic metabolism can lead to an accumulation of lactic acid and slowed conduction velocity to muscle fibers, resulting in muscle fatigue, reduced tension development, and eventual inability to hold a contraction (Basmajian & DeLuca, 1985). Persons with poor neuromuscular endurance will experience muscle fatigue sooner than those with good neuromuscular endurance.

Static endurance refers to the measure of sustained contractions. Isometric testing times how long an individual can maintain the tension of a maximum voluntary contraction via strain gauges, dynamometers, and some isokinetic equipment. Normally, a person can hold 25% MVC for 5 to 6 minutes, 50% MVC for 1 to 2 minutes, and 100% MVC only momentarily (Dehn & Mullins, 1977; Minor, 1991). Persons being tested should talk while doing an isometric contraction to preclude breath holding and a significant increase in blood pressure or additional stress to the cardiopulmonary system.

Clinical Functional Endurance

Perhaps the most pertinent clinical information regarding muscular endurance comes from monitoring client progress through a treatment program as opposed to comparing scores to population norms. One can evaluate and quantify endurance performance by applying the principles of the timed test of repetitions at a submaximal workload. Another method is to time how long a client can participate in such activities of daily living such as dressing or light homemaking before requiring a rest. Another method that is clinically applicable to evaluating changes in activity tolerance is to monitor the client's perception of how hard he/she is working or how tired he/she is after a given amount of time at a specified workload. One accepted such scale is the Borg Scale of Rating of Perceived Exertion (RPE) which ranges from "no work at all" (0 on the scale) to "very very heavy work" (10 on the scale) (Brannon, Foley, Starr, & Black, 1993; Minor, 1991).

GROSS COORDINATION

Many types of lesions can produce disturbances of coordination. Cerebellar lesions, muscle or peripheral nerve disease or injury, lesions of the posterior column of the spinal cord, and lesions of the frontal or post central cortex can all cause incoordination.

Cerebellar Dysfunction

Types of cerebellar dysfunction and methods of evaluating them are as follows:

Intention Tremor: Intention tremor occurs during voluntary movement, is less apparent or absent during rest, and intensifies at the termination of the movement. To test for this, the therapist can ask the client to alternately touch his own nose and then the therapist's finger, held in front of the client in various positions. Tremor can also be observed during performance of daily activities, or during the finger to finger test. Similar to the finger to nose test, the client is asked to touch one of the examiner's fingers, then another held a distance away. Distance and target points are changed as the therapist notes tremor level, speed of response, and success rate.

Dysdiadochokinesia: Dysdiadochokinesia is a decreased ability to perform rapid alternating movements smoothly. Tests include having the client supinate and pronate the forearm, flex and extend the elbow, or grasp and release. Other tests include alternate rotation of fully extended arms or tapping the table with extended fingers. Tests are performed bilaterally. The number of alternations within a given time period and any differences between extremities are noted.

Dysmetria: Dysmetria is the inability to control muscle length which results in overshooting or pointing past an object. The finger to nose or finger to finger test are used to evaluate this. Functionally, a client may hit himself in the face with a comb in an attempt to comb his hair, or overshoot and miss picking up the comb from the nightstand.

Dyssynergia: Dyssynergia is a decomposition of movement. The lack of synergistic action between agonists and antagonists produces jerky movements. Dyssynergia can be observed in the alternating movement, finger to nose, and finger to finger tests.

Ataxic Gait: Ataxic gait is often unsteady and wide-based; clients with this gait show a tendency to veer or fall to the side of the lesion. The therapist can observe the client walking or ask the client to walk and turn quickly or walk heel to toe along a straight line.

Rebound Phenomenon of Holmes: Rebound Phenomenon of Holmes is a lack of a "check reflex" to stop a motion to avoid striking something in the path of motion. To test, the examiner resists the elbow flexion at the forearm and unexpectedly releases the resistance; the client's hand may hit his or her own chest, shoulder, or face if he or she is unable to check the motion.

Hypotonia: Hypotonia is decreased muscle tone and decreased resistance to passive movement due to the loss of the cerebellum's facilitory influence on the stretch reflex. The therapist can observe hypotonia clinically and perform a quick stretch.

Posterior Column Dysfunction

Types posterior column dysfunction and methods of evaluating them are as follows:

Ataxia: In this case the wide-based gait results from loss of proprioception. The client's ability to self-correct if he or she visually compensates as he or she watches the floor and placement of the feet differentiates posterior column from cerebellar dysfunction.

Romberg Sign: Romberg Sign is the inability to maintain standing balance with feet together and eyes closed. In posterior column deficit, dysmetria in the finger to nose test is exacerbated with the eyes closed.

Basal Ganglia Dysfunction

Types basal ganglia dysfunction and methods of evaluating them are as follows:

Athetosis: Athetosis is a movement disorder characterized by slow, writhing, twisting, continuous, and involuntary movements, particularly of the neck, face, and extremities. These movements are not present during sleep. Muscles may have either increased or decreased tone. The therapist should note proximal or distal involvement, involved extremities, pattern of motions and what stimuli increase or decrease the abnormal movements.

Dystonia: Dystonia is a form of athetosis that causes twisting movements of the trunk and proximal muscles of the extremities, distorted postures, and torsion spasms.

Chorea: Choreiform movements are irregular, purposeless, coarse, quick, jerky, and dysrhythmic. Muscles are hypotonic. Chorea may occur in sleep.

Hemiballism: Hemiballism is a rare, unilateral chorea that is a violent, forceful, sudden flinging movements of the extremities on one side of the body.

Tremors at Rest: Resting tremors stop at the initiation of voluntary movement but resume during the holding phase of a motor task, particularly when the client is tired or attention is diverted. An example is the pill-rolling tremor seen in Parkinsonism.

Bradykinesia: Bradykinesia means poverty of movement. Automatic movements such as arm swinging during gait and facial expressions are diminished (Mathiowetz & Haugen, 1995; Smith, 1993; Undzis et al., 1996).

POSTURAL CONTROL

Before evaluation of postural control, one needs to do an examination of posture. Posture is a composite of the positions of all the joints of the body at any given time. It is the static position assumed by any body part of by the body in general that requires muscular effort (Brooks, 1986; Farber, 1991a,b; Kendall et al., 1993). Kinesiologically, one needs to evaluate spinal alignment and curves, pelvis, trunk, head/neck, and upper extremity posture alone and in relation to each other in positions of standing, sitting, and lying down if appropriate. Good body alignment occurs when the center of gravity of each body segment is located over the supporting base of the body. Structural problems and muscle strength deficits/imbalances can have a mechanical effect on postural control.

Postural control, or balance, refers to the ability to maintain the center of body mass or a body part over a stable or moving base of support (Crutchfield, Shumway-Cook, & Horak, 1989). There are several prerequisites for "normal" internal postural control. Clients need to be able to:

1) Produce movement through adequate range of motion in the trunk and extremities.
2) Differentiate body parts from one another (for example, rotate the head independently of the shoulders).
3) Stop and hold movement at mid-range of motion in order to stabilize against gravity. This is critical for transitional movement.
4) Distribute normal postural tone in the body segments to support movement.
5) Function symmetrically (Gilfoyle, Grady & Moore, 1981).

One difficulty in identifying the specific determinants of balance deficits is that balance behavior can be influenced by the somatosensory (proprioceptive, cutaneous, and joint), visual, and vestibular systems. Clients may show deficits in balance control during expected and unexpected perturbations, voluntary postural adjustments, or postural adjustments preceding voluntary limb movements. Valid conclusions about balance dysfunction require tests that differentiate between conditions that modify sensory inputs (Difablo & Badke, 1990).

The therapist should note clinical observations regarding the clients ability to acquire and maintain the following developmental positions: prone, supine, sitting, crawling, standing, and walking, noting automatic responses in sagittal, frontal, and transverse body planes. Balance during various functional activities, such as reaching in the kitchen, tying shoes and bathing should be noted as well. Lastly, there are several clinical assessment tools that evaluate postural control (Table E-10).

FINE COORDINATION/DEXTERITY

There are several standardized tests which evaluate aspects of dexterity such as speed of object manipulation, accuracy of movement, grasp and release, prehension patterns, writing skills, and hand posture

TABLE E-10	POSTURAL CONTROL ASSESSMENTS	
Assessment	**Description**	**Source**
Berg Balance Scale	Client asked to complete 14 different tasks. Each task is scored using a 4-point scale.	Berg, Wood-Dauphinee, & Williams, 1989
Functional Reach	Measures the distance between the anatomical reach and the maximal reach without slipping.	Duncan, Weiner, Chandler & Studenski, 1990
Physical Performance Test	Measures physical capabilities of older adults for functional activities. Seven of nine items are related to static and dynamic balance (e.g., donning & doffing a jacket, putting a book on a high shelf). Two items are related to writing and eating.	Reuben & Siu, 1990
Timed "Up and Go" Test (TU&GT)	Measures the time it takes for an older adult to stand up from a standard armchair, walk a short distance, turn, return to the chair and sit down.	Podsiadlo & Richardson, 1991
Tinetti's Balance and Gait Evaluation	Client is asked to do a variety of tasks such as move from sitting to standing, ambulate. Has high predictive validity for frail elderly at risk for falls.	Tinetti, 1986

Derived from Whitney, Poole, and Cass (1998) and Kohlmeyer, K. (1998). Evaluation of sensory and neuromuscular performance components. In M. E. Neistadt & E. B. Crepeau (Eds.), *Willard & Spackman's occupational therapy* (9th ed.) (pp. 223–260). Philadelphia: Lippincott, p. 258. Reprinted from latter, with permission.

(Farber, 1991a,b; Mathiowetz & Haugen, 1995; Smith, 1993; Undzis et al., 1996). These tests are usually administered with the individual sitting with the arm supported. However, it is important to observe fine motor functioning in a variety of positions with the arm supported and unsupported as they occur in activities of daily living.

Functional tasks such as buttoning, using scissors, handling coins, and writing should be observed for the ease, accuracy, and timing of performance. The tests listed in Table E-11 can be used to specifically

TABLE E-11	FINE MOTOR COORDINATION TESTS	
Assessment	**Description**	**Source**
Box and Block Test (Mathiowetz, Volland, Kashman, & Weber, 1985)	Tests manual dexterity. Normed for children 7–9 years old, adults and adults with neuromuscular involvement. Picking up one block at a time and placing it in attached compartment.	Sammons Preston P.O. Box 5071 Bolingbrook, IL 60440-5071 1-800-547-4333
Crawford Small Parts Dexterity Test	Measures eye-hand coordination and manipulation of small hand tools. Designed for teenagers and adults. Pins, collars, screws, tweezers, screwdriver. Examinee is timed on tasks such as inserting pen in hole in metal plate with tweezers, covering with collar, threading screws.	Psychological Corporation 304 East 45th St., New York, NY 10017
Jebsen-Taylor Hand Function Test (Jebsen, Taylor, Trieschmann, Trotter, & Howard, 1969)	Evaluates functional capabilities. Sub-tests include writing, card-turning, picking up small objects, simulated feeding, stacking checkers, picking up light and heavy objects.	Sammons Preston P.O. Box 5071 Bolingbrook, IL 60440-5071 1-800-547-4333
Minnesota Rate of Manipulation Test	Measures dexterity. Placing, turning, displacing, one-hand turning and placing and two-hand turning, and placing round blocks.	American Guidance Service Publishers Bldg. Circle Pines, MN 55014; Sammons Preston P.O. Box 5071 Bolingbrook, IL 60440-5071 1-800-547-4333

continued

APPENDIX E

TABLE E-11	FINE MOTOR COORDINATION TESTS (CONTINUED)

Assessment	Description	Source
Nine Hole Peg Test of Fine Motor Coordination (Mathiowetz, Weber, Kashman, & Volland, 1985)	Measures fine dexterity. Normed for adults over 20 years. Timed score to place nine 1 1/4" pegs in a 5×5" board and remove them.	Sammons Preston P.O. Box 5071 Bolingbrook, IL 60440-5071 1-800-547-4333
O'Connor Finger and Tweezer Dexterity Tests	Measures dexterity. Normed for adults. Picking up pins 1" long, I/16" diameter with fingers (Finger Dexterity) or with tweezers (Tweezer Dexterity) and placing in 10 rows of 10 holes. Timed test.	Sammons Preston P.O. Box 5071 Bolingbrook, IL 60440-5071 1-800-547-4333; Smith+Nephew One Quality Drive, P.O. Box 1005 Germantown, WI 53022-8205 1-800-545-8633
Purdue Pegboard Test	Measures movements of arms, hands, fingers and fingertip dexterity. Normed for adults and children 5 years to 15 years, 11 months. Placing pins in pegboard; assembly of pins, washers and collars.	Science Research Assoc. 259 E. Erie St. Chicago, IL 60611; Sammons Preston P.O. Box 5071 Bolingbrook, IL 60440-5071 1-800-547-4333
The Grooved Pegboard Test	Measures eye-hand coordination and finger dexterity. Placing grooved pegs in 25 hole pegbaord, in various random positions.	Lafayette Instrument Co., P.O. Box 5729 Lafayette, IN 47903; Sammons Preston P.O. Box 5071 Bolingbrook, IL 60440-5071 1-800-547-4333

(Farber, 1991, a, b; Mathiowetz & Haugen, 1995; Smith, 1993; Undzis et al., 1996)
Derived and reprinted with permission from Kohlmeyer, K. (1998). Evaluation of sensory and neuromuscular performance components. In M. E. Neistadt & E. B. Crepeau (Eds.), *Willard & Spackman's occupational therapy* (9th ed.) (pp. 223–260). Philadelphia: Lippincott, p. 259.

identify as well as monitor progress with dexterity difficulties in a more standardized fashion.

Recording Results

Observation of functional abilities can be recorded directly on the initial evaluation. Results of standardized tests should be recorded per direction of each test.

Interpreting Results

Irregularity in rate of movement, excessive force, incorrect sequencing, and sudden corrective movements may indicate problems with coordination. Scores on standardized dexterity tests below norms also signal fine motor coordination problems. Determining the root(s) of the problem leads to a treatment plan. Several considerations should include sensory, specifically proprioceptive deficits, problems with body scheme, coordination of agonist/antagonist muscles, and ability to accurately judge space; cerebellar, spinal cord, posterior column, frontal, and post central cerebral cortex lesions also affect coordination. Again, the focus of treatment should be the functional implications of the performance deficit (Undzis et al., 1996).

With the exception of ordering information, unless otherwise noted, the information in this appendix has been modified and reprinted with permission from: Kohlmeyer, K. (1998). Evaluation of sensory and neuromuscular performance components. In M. E. Neistadt & E. B. Crepeau (eds.), Willard & Spackman's occupational therapy (9th ed.), pp. 223–260. Philadelphia: Lippincott.

APPENDIX E

F

PSYCHOSOCIAL SKILLS ASSESSMENTS

With the exception of ordering information, unless otherwise noted, the information in this appendix has been modified and reprinted with permission from: Henry, A. (1998). The interview process in occupational therapy. In M.E. Neistadt & E.B. Crepeau (Eds.), *Willard & Spackman's Occupational Therapy* (pp.155–168). Philadelphia: Lippincott.

ALLEN COGNITIVE LEVEL TEST-90 (ACLS-90)

Purpose

The ACLS-90 (Allen, 1996) is the latest version of the Allen Cognitive Level Test (ACL). The ACLS-90 was designed to determine a client's cognitive level according to the Cognitive Disabilities Model (CDM) (Allen, 1985; Allen, Earhart, & Blue, 1992). The CDM is a schema of 7 levels to describe cognitive abilities ranging from normal (Level 6) to coma (Level 0). The behaviors associated with Levels 0–5 are further delineated by decimal levels; Level 1 (coma) has only one decimal level, Levels 2–5 have 5 decimal levels each. The ACLS-90 is most appropriate to screen for cognitive difficulties for clients at Levels 3–5 (Allen, 1992).

Description

The ACLS-90 is a leather lacing task. Clients are assigned a cognitive level score from 3.0 to 5.8 based on their ability to perform three progressively difficult leather lacing stitches—sewing, whip, and single cordovan (Henry et al., 1998; Allen, 1992). A larger version is available (Larger Allen Cognitive Screen) for clients with visual impairments (Allen, 1998).

Psychometric Properties

Several studies have shown various versions of the ACL to have high interrater reliability. In a more recent study the interrater reliability of the ACLS-90 was 0.92 (Henry et al., 1998). Several studies have also established the validity of the ACL by showing that ACL scores significantly correlate with measures of other cognitive abilities, social skills, and symptomatology, and without psychiatric disorders. A more recent study showed ACL-90 scores to be strongly related to discharge living situations and able to discriminate between clients with and without psychosis (Henry et al., 1998).

Ordering Information

Contact S & S Worldwide, Norwich Ave., Colchester, CT; 1-800-243-9232; www.sns.wwide.com

ROLE ACTIVITY PERFORMANCE SCALE (RAPS)

Purpose

The RAPS (Good-Ellis, Fine, Spencer & DiVittis, 1987) was designed to assess an individual's history of role performance over a period of up to 18 months. Developed for use with adult psychiatric patients, the RAPS was designed to facilitate treatment planning and to be used as a research tool in treatment outcome studies (Good-Ellis, et al., 1987).

Description

The RAPS covers role performance in 12 areas: work/work equivalent, education, home management, family relationships, mate relationships, parental role, social relationships, leisure activities, self-management, health care, hygiene and appearance, and health care role. The interviewer covers only those role areas that are relevant. Unlike interviews which rely only on client self-report, the RAPS allows for data to be gathered from a variety of other sources, including family members, the medical record, and the treatment team. Prior to the interview, the interviewer asks the client to complete a self-report questionnaire, reviews the medical record for pertinent data, and contacts other sources in order to determine which role areas should be covered during the interview. A set of recommended question has been developed for each role area, and the format of the questions is similar across role areas (Good-Ellis, et al., 1987).

Each relevant role area is rated utilizing a 6-point scale, with a score of "1" denoting excellent or good role performance, and "6" indicating an inability to function in the role (Good-Ellis, et al., 1987). In addition, because the RAPS is intended to evaluate role functioning over time, separate ratings in each role area are made retrospectively on a monthly basis up to 18 months prior to the interview. This retrospective rating allows for scores reflecting the individual's performance within each role over time, as well as a total score reflecting the individual's performance across roles over time (Good-Ellis, et al., 1987). A manual detailing the administration and scoring of the RAPS is currently in production (Good-Ellis, personal communication, May, 1996).

Method

The RAPS is a semi-structured interview and rating procedure.

Psychometric Properties

Several studies have shown the RAPS to have good interrater reliability (Good-Ellis et al., 1987), concurrent validity (Good-Ellis et al., 1987) and criterion-related validity (Good-Ellis et al., 1986; Good-Ellis et al., 1987).

Ordering Information

Contact Susan Fine, MA, OTR, FAOTA; 201 E. 79th Street; New York, NY 10021

THE ASSESSMENT OF OCCUPATIONAL FUNCTIONING (AOF)

Purpose

The AOF (Watts, Brollier, Bauer & Schmidt, 1988b) is also based on the MOHO. The AOF was initially developed as a screening tool for use with either physically or psychiatrically disabled clients in long-term care settings. However, the most recent version, published in Occupational Therapy in Mental Health (Watts, et al., 1988b), has been revised to be appropriate for use in other settings.

Description

The AOF is a semi-structured interview with 23 questions which tap the client's current functioning consistent with MOHO constructs.

The AOF rating scale consists of 20 items, with 3–4 items comprising each of six subscales: values, personal causation, interests, roles, habits, and skills. Each item poses a question (e.g., "Does this person routinely pursue his/her interests?"), which is then rated from 5 ("very highly") to 1 ("very little"). All 20 items may be summed for a total score (Watts, et al., 1988b).

Method

The AOF is a semi-structured interview.

Psychometric Properties

The original version of the AOF has both interrater and test-retest reliability (Watts et al., 1986). No reliability data on the most recent revised version of the AOF rating scale have been reported. Studies have shown both the original and revised versions of the AOF to have concurrent validity (Brollier et al., 1988; Watts, Brollier, Bauer, & Schmidt, 1988a). Moreover, the AOF was found to discriminate between healthy community subjects and subjects in institutions 94% of the time (Watts et al., 1986).

Ordering Information

Available in: Watts, J. H., Brollier, C., Bauer, D., & Schmidt, W. (1988b). The assessment of occupational functioning: The second revision. *Occupational Therapy in Mental Health, 8*(4), 7–27.

THE OCCUPATIONAL CASE ANALYSIS AND INTERVIEW RATING SCALE (OCAIRS)

Purpose

The OCAIRS (Kaplan & Kielhofner, 1989) was designed for use in short-term adult psychiatric settings. It was the first interview procedure specifically designed to reflect the Model of Human Occupation (MOHO) (Kielhofner, 1985, 1995) perspective.

Description

The OCAIRS includes approximately 38 recommended questions which are designed to address MOHO components. A 5-point rating scale, with 14 items, accompanies the interview. The items include personal causation, values and goals, interests, roles, habits, skills, output, physical environment, social environment, feedback, dynamic (gestalt functioning), historical (life history pattern), contextual (environmental influence) and system trajectory (occupational prognosis). The client's functioning relative to each item is rated from adaptive (5) to maladaptive (1).

Method

The OCAIRS is a semi-structured interview.

Psychometric Properties

Several studies have established the interrater reliability and concurrent validity of the OCAIRS (Brollier, Watts, Bauer & Schmidt, 1988; Kaplan & Kielhofner, 1989; Watts et al., 1988a).

Ordering Information

A detailed training manual on the administration and interpretation of the OCAIRS is available: Kaplan, K., & Kielhofner, G. (1989). Occupational case analysis interview and rating scale. Thorofare, NJ: Slack, Inc. [SLACK Inc.; 6900 Grove Road; Thorofare, NJ 08086; 1-800-257-8290; FAX (609) 853-5991; www.slackinc.com]

APPENDIX F

THE OCCUPATIONAL PERFORMANCE HISTORY INTERVIEW II (OPHI II)

Purpose

The OPHI-II (Kielhofner, Mallinson, Crawford, Nowak, Rigby, Henry, & Walens, 1998) was designed to gather information about a client's occupational history related to work, play, and daily living activities (Henry & Mallinson, 1999). It is appropriate for adults who can reflect on and discuss their life history.

Description

The OPHI II consists of three parts administered in the following order: (a) a semi-structured interview, (b) rating scales, and (c) a life history narrative. The semi-structured interview contains interview questions, with alternatives, in five thematic areas that reflect the theoretical constructs of the Model of Human Occupation: (a) activity/occupational choices, (b) critical life events, (c) daily routine, (d) occupational roles, (e) occupational behavior settings. Therapists can cover the thematic areas in any sequence or can move back and forth between areas. The three rating scales which are applied to the information derived from the semi-structured interview are: (a) the Occupational Identity Scale (11 items), (b) the Occupational Competence Scale (9 items), and (c) the Occupational Behavior Settings Scale (9 items). The rating scales use a four-point scale to indicate a client's level of adaptation for each item. The life history narrative is completed by filling out the Life History Form. This form requests a time line representing the client's life and a brief narrative of the client's life history. The OPHI II can be administered in 45–60 minutes and so is most appropriate in settings where the therapist anticipates seeing the client for a course of intervention (Henry & Mallinson, 1999)

Method

The OPHI II is a semi-structured interview.

Psychometric Properties

Rasch analysis of the three rating scales in a study involving 64 occupational therapists and 44 clients from 4 countries (Australia, Belgium, Finland, United States) indicated high reliability for each scale (0.90–0.96) and high rater consistency. Construct validity was supported by the fact that all items fit for each scale (Henry & Mallinson, 1999).

Ordering Information

AOTA Products; P.O. Box 64949; Baltimore, MD 21264-4949; 1-800-SAY-AOTA for AOTA members; (301) 652-AOTA (2682) for non-members

G

DISCHARGE SITUATION ASSESSMENTS

The following discharge situation assessments have been reprinted, with permission from Cedar Sinai Medical Center, 8700 Beverly Boulevard, Box 48750, Los Angeles, CA 90048-0750.

CEDARS-SINAI MEDICAL CENTER
ACUTE REHABILITATION IN-PATIENT UNIT

File _____

PATIENT I.D.

PRE-HOME ASSESSMENT

DATE	PATIENT NAME		TELEPHONE NUMBER
ADDRESS			THERAPIST'S NAME
TYPE OF RESIDENCE (i.e., house, apt., condo, etc.)	CONTACT PERSON		TELEPHONE NUMBER

ENTRANCE: (used most)

_____ Front   Elevator: (Width, Threshold) _____
_____ Side   Doorway Width (s): _____
_____ Back   Stairs (How many, Height of step) _____
_____ Garage   Railing (s): (which side) _____
                  Ramp (s): ❐ Yes ❐ No
                  Threshold Height: _____
                  Hazards: (i.e. rug/mat, cords, etc.) _____

LIVING AREA:

Doorway Width(s): _____ Threshold: ❐ Yes ❐ No
Carpeting: ❐ Yes ❐ No   What type? _____
Couch/Seat Height: (most used) _____
   armrests: ❐ Yes ❐ No
Hazards: (telephone/light cords, torn carpet, throw rugs, etc.)
_____

KITCHEN/DINING ROOM:

Doorway Width(s): _____ Threshold: ❐ Yes ❐ No
Chair Height: ❐ With Arms ❐ Without Arms
Table Height: _____
Counter Height: _____

BEDROOM:

Doorway Width(s): _____ Threshold: ❐ Yes ❐ No
Bed Height/Firmness/Size: _____
Side of Bed Preferred for Sleeping: _____
Closet Height: _____
Dresser Drawers Height: _____
Carpeting: _____
Hazards: _____
Length & Width of Pathway: _____

Form No. 4900 (8/93)

FIGURE G-1.   Pre-Home Assessment From Cedars-Sinai Medical Center.
Reprinted with permission of Cedars-Sinai Medical Center.

NAME OF PATIENT (LAST NAME, FIRST)	HOSPITAL I.D. NUMBER

BATHROOM: (used most)

Doorway Width(s): _____ Threshold: ☐ Yes ☐ No

Tub:

    Curtain or Doors _____

    Height Outside _____

    Height Inside _____

    Width Inside _____

How many walls surround tub? (circle one)

TUB	TUB	TUB	TUB

Shower Stall:

    Door: Sliding or Hinge _____

        Direction Door Swings (Left/Right) _____

    Step Height: Inside _____

             Outside _____

Toilet Height: _____

Basin Height: _____

EQUIPMENT AVAILABLE FOR HOME USE:

_____ Rubber mat

_____ Shower chair (describe) _____

_____ Grab bars

_____ Raised Toilet seat

_____ Other

SAFETY HAZARDS:

_____ Obstructions	_____ Highly waxed floors
_____ Sharp edged furniture	_____ Indoor stair cases
_____ Throw rugs	_____ No bath mat or bathstrips
_____ Loose wires/telephone	_____ Other
_____ Stairs need repair	_____ Poor lighting

PLEASE LIST ANY QUESTIONS YOU MAY HAVE:

APPENDIX G

CEDARS-SINAI MEDICAL CENTER
ACUTE REHABILITATION IN-PATIENT UNIT
HOME ASSESSMENT REPORT

PATIENT I.D.

DATE

PATIENT DIAGNOSIS

ADDRESS

TELEPHONE NUMBER

DESTINATION

TYPE OF RESIDENCE

Patient Present for Visit: ☐ Yes ☐ No   Level of Mobility: _____

Family/Attendant Present: ☐ Yes ☐ No   Specify: _____

ENTRANCE:
☐ Front
☐ Side
☐ Back
☐ Garage

Elevator: (Width, Threshold) _____

Doorway Width(s): _____

Stairs (# & Hgt): _____

Railing(s): _____

Ramp(s): _____

Threshold: _____

Hazards: _____

DIAGRAMS, ROOMS NOT ALREADY ADDRESSED:

LIVING AREA:

Doorway Width(s): _____

Carpeting: _____

Couch/Seat Height: _____

Hazards: _____
(Telephone/Light Cords, Torn Carpet, Throw Rugs)

KITCHEN:

Doorway Width(s): _____

Chair Height: _____
(Kitchen/Dining Room)

Hazards: _____

BATHROOM:

Doorway Width(s): _____

Tub/Shower: _____
(Rim Width, Curtain/Doors, Step Hgt/Width, Tub Width)

Toilet Hgt/Access: _____

Basin Hgt/Access: _____

BEDROOM:

Doorway Width(s): _____

Bed Hgt/Firmness: _____

Closet Hgt/Access: _____

Dresser Drawers Hgt/Access: _____

Carpeting: _____

Hazards: _____

Therapist: _____

Form No. 222 Rev. 3/92

FIGURE G-2. Home Assessment From Cedars-Sinai Medical Center. Reprinted with permission of Cedars-Sinai Medical Center.

NAME OF PATIENT (LAST NAME, FIRST NAME, MIDDLE INITIAL)	HOSPITAL I.D. NUMBER

COMMENTS/RECOMMENDATIONS: _____

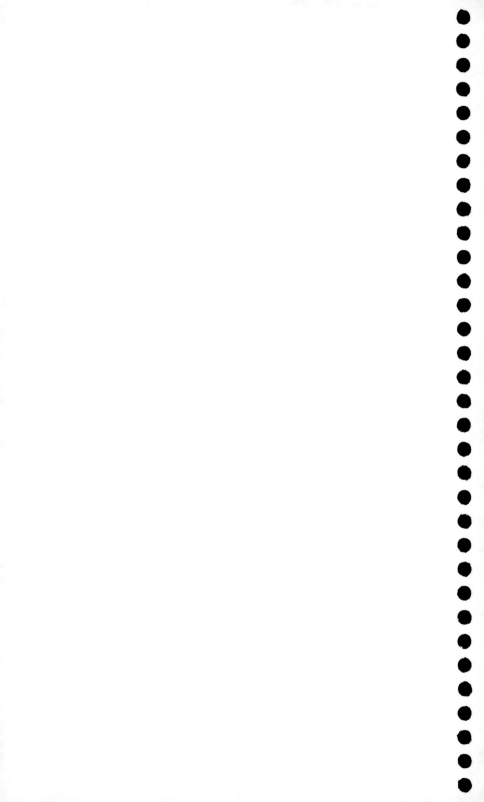

H
UNIFORM TERMINOLOGY

This is an official document of The American Occupational Therapy Association (AOTA). This document is intended to provide a generic outline of the domain of concern of occupational therapy and is designed to create common terminology for the profession and to capture the essence of occupational therapy succinctly for others.

It is recognized that the phenomena that constitute the profession's domain of concern can be categorized, and labeled, in a number of different ways. This document is not meant to limit those in the field, formulating theories or frames of reference, who may wish to combine or refine particular constructs. It is also not meant to limit those who would like to conceptualize the profession's domain of concern in a different manner.

INTRODUCTION

The first edition of Uniform Terminology was approved and published in 1979 (AOTA, 1979). In 1989, Uniform Terminology for Occupational Therapy—Second Edition (AOTA, 1989) was approved and published. The second document presented an organized structure for understanding the areas of practice for the profession of occupational therapy. The document outlined two domains. Performance areas (activities of daily living [ADL], work and productive activities, and play or leisure) include activities that the occupational therapy practitioner emphasizes when determining functional abilities (occupational therapy practitioner refers to both registered occupational therapists and certified occupational therapy assistants). Performance components (sensorimotor, cognitive, psychosocial, and

Reprint of: American Occupational Therapy Association (1994). Uniform terminology for occupational therapy—3rd edition. *American Journal of Occupational Therapy, 48,* 1047–1054, with permission.

psychological aspects) are the elements of performance that occupational therapists assess and, when needed, in which they intervene for improved performance.

This third edition has been further expanded to reflect current practice and to incorporate contextual aspects of performance. Performance areas, performance components, and performance contexts are the parameters of occupational therapy's domain of concern. Performance areas are broad categories of human activity that are typically part of daily life. They are activities of daily living, work and productive activities, and play or leisure activities. Performance components are fundamental human abilities that—to varying degrees and in differing combinations—are required for successful engagement in performance areas. These components are sensorimotor, cognitive, psychosocial, and psychological. Performance contexts are situations or factors that influence an individual's engagement in desired and/or required performance areas. Performance contexts consist of temporal aspects (chronological age, developmental age, place in the life cycle, and health status) and environmental aspects (physical, social, and cultural considerations). There is an interactive relationship among performance areas, performance components, and performance contexts. Function in performance areas is the ultimate concern of occupational therapy, with performance components considered as they relate to participation in performance areas. Performance areas and performance components are always viewed within performance contexts. Performance contexts are taken into consideration when determining function and dysfunction relative to performance areas and performance components, and in planning intervention. For example, the occupational therapist does not evaluate strength (a performance component) in isolation. Strength is considered as it affects necessary or desired tasks (performance areas). If the individual is interested in homemaking, the occupational therapy practitioner would consider the interaction of strength with homemaking tasks. Strengthening could be addressed through kitchen activities, such as cooking and putting groceries away. In some cases, the practitioner would employ an adaptive approach and recommend that the family switch from heavy stoneware to lighter-weight dishes, or use lighter-weight pots on the stove to enable the individual to make dinner safely without becoming fatigued or compromising safety.

Occupational therapy assessment involves examining performance areas, performance components, and performance contexts. Intervention may be directed toward elements of performance areas (e.g., dressing, vocational exploration), performance components (e.g., endurance, problem solving), or the environment aspects of performance contexts. In the latter case, the physical and/or social environment may be altered or augmented to improve and/or maintain function. After identifying the performance areas the individual wishes or needs to address, the occupational therapist assesses the features of the environments in which the tasks will be performed. If an individual's job requires cooking in a restaurant as opposed to leisure cooking at home, the occupational therapy practitioner faces several challenges to enable the individual's success in different environments. Therefore, the third critical aspect of performance is the performance context, the features of the environment that affect the person's ability to engage in functional activities.

This document categorizes specific activities in each of the performance areas (ADL, work and productive activities, play or leisure). This categorization is based on what is considered "typical," and is not meant to imply that a particular individual characterizes personal activities in the same manner as someone else. Occupational therapy practitioners embrace individual differences, and so would document the unique pattern of the individual being served, rather than forcing the "typical" pattern on him or her and family. For example, because of experience or culture, a particular individual might think of home management as an ADL task rather than "work and productive activities" (current listing). Socialization might be considered part of a play or leisure activity instead of its current listing as part of "activities of daily living," because of life experience or cultural heritage.

EXAMPLES OF USE IN PRACTICE

Uniform Terminology—Third Edition defines occupational therapy's domain of concern, which includes performance areas, performance components, and performance contexts. While this document may be used by occupational therapy practitioners in a number of different areas (e.g., practice, documentation, charge systems, education, program development, marketing, research, disability classifications, and regulations), it focuses on the use of uniform terminology in practice. This document is not intended to define specific occupational therapy programs or specific occupational therapy interventions. Examples of how performance areas, performance components, and performance contexts translate into practice are provided below.

- An individual who is injured on the job may have the potential to return to work and productive activities, which is a performance area. In order to achieve the outcome of returning to work and productive activities, the individual may need to address specific performance components, such as strength, endurance, soft tissue integrity, time management, and the physical features of performance contexts, like structures and objects in his or her environment. The occupational therapy practitioner, in collaboration with the individual and other members of the vocational team, uses planned interventions to achieve the desired outcome. These interventions may include activities such as an exercise program, body mechanics instruction, and job site modifications, all of which may be provided in a work-hardening program.

- An elderly individual recovering from a cerebrovascular accident may wish to live in a community setting, which combines the performance areas of ADL with work and productive activities. In order to achieve the outcome of community living, the individual may need to address specific performance components, such as muscle tone, gross motor coordination, postural control, and self-management. It is also necessary to consider the sociocultural and physical features of performance contexts, such as support available from other persons, and adaptations of structures and objects within the environment. The occupational therapy practitioner, in cooperation with the team, utilizes planned interventions to achieve the desired outcome. Interventions may include neuromuscular facilitation, practice of object manipulation, and instruction in the use of adaptive equipment and home safety equipment. The practitioner and individual also pursue the selection and training of a personal assistant to ensure the completion of ADL tasks. These interventions may be provided in a comprehensive inpatient rehabilitation unit.

- A child with learning disabilities is required to perform educational activities within a public school setting. Engaging in educational activities is considered the performance area of work and productive activities for this child. To achieve the educational outcome of efficient and effective completion of written classroom work, the child may need to address specific performance components. These include sensory processing, perceptual skills, postural control, motor skills, and the physical features of performance contexts, such as objects (e.g., desk, chair) in the environment. In cooperation with the team, occupational therapy interventions may include activities like adapting the student's seating in the classroom to improve postural control and stability, and practicing motor control and coordination. This program could be developed by an occupational therapist and supported by school district personnel.

- The parents of an infant with cerebral palsy may ask to facilitate the child's involvement in the performance areas of activities of daily living and play. Subsequent to assessment, the therapist identifies specific performance components, such as sensory awareness and neuromuscular control. The practitioner also addresses the physical and cultural features of performance contexts. In collaboration with the parents, occupational therapy interventions may include activities such as seating and positioning for play, neuromuscular facilitation techniques to enable eating, facilitating parent skills in caring for and playing with their infant, and modifying the play space for accessibility. These interventions may be provided in a home-based occupational therapy program.

- An adult with schizophrenia may need and want to live independently in the community, which represents the performance areas of activities of daily living, work and productive activities, and leisure activities. The specific performance categories may be medication routine, functional mobility, home management, vocational exploration, play or leisure performance, and social interaction. In order to achieve the outcome of living independently, the individual may need to address specific performance components, such as topographical orientation; memory; categorization; problem solving; interests; social conduct; time management; and sociocultural features of performance contexts, such as social factors (e.g., influence of family and friends) and roles. The occupational therapy practitioner, in cooperation with the team, utilizes planned interventions to achieve the desired outcome. Interventions may include activities such as training in the use of public transportation, instruction in budgeting skills, selection and participation in social activities, instruction in social conduct, and participation in community reintegration activities. These interventions may be provided in a community-based mental health program.

- An individual with a history of substance abuse may need to reestablish family roles and responsibilities, which represent the performance areas of activities of daily living, work and productive activities, and leisure activities. In order to achieve the outcome of family participation, the individual may need to address the performance components of roles; values; social conduct; self-expression; coping skills; self-control; and the sociocultural features of performance contexts, such as custom, behavior, rules, and rituals. The occupational therapy practitioner, in cooperation with the team, utilizes planned interventions to achieve the desired outcomes. Interventions may include roles and values exercises, instruction in stress management techniques, identification of family roles and activities, and support to develop family leisure routines. These interventions may be provided in an inpatient acute care unit.

APPENDIX H

PERSON–ACTIVITY–ENVIRONMENT FIT

Person–activity–environment fit refers to the match among the skills and abilities of the individual; the demands of the activity; and the characteristics of the physical, social, and cultural environments. It is the interaction among the performance areas, performance components, and performance contexts that is important and determines the success of the performance. When occupational therapy practitioners provide services, they attend to all of these aspects of performance and the interaction among them. They also attend to each individual's unique personal history. The personal history includes one's skills and abilities (performance components), the past performance of specific life tasks (performance areas), and experience within particular environments (performance contexts). In addition to personal history, anticipated life tasks and role demands influence performance.

When considering the person–activity–environment fit, variables such as novelty, importance, motivation, activity tolerance, and quality are salient. Situations range from those that are completely familiar to those that are novel and have never been experienced. Both the novelty and familiarity within a situation contribute to the overall task performance. In each situation, there is an optimal level of novelty that engages the individual sufficiently and provides enough information to perform the task. When too little novelty is present, the individual may miss cues and opportunities to perform. When too much novelty is present, the individual may become confused and distracted, inhibiting effective task performance.

Humans determine that some stimuli and situations are more meaningful than others. Individuals perform tasks they deem important. It is critical to identify what the individual wants or needs to do when planning interventions.

The level of motivation an individual demonstrates to perform a particular task is determined by both internal and external factors. An individual's biobehavioral state (e.g., amount of rest, arousal, tension) contributes to the potential to be responsive. The features of the social and physical environments (e.g., persons in the room, noise level) provide information that is either adequate or inadequate to produce a motivated state.

Activity tolerance is the individual's ability to sustain a purposeful activity over time. Individuals must not only select, initiate, and terminate activities, but they must also attend to a task for the needed length of time to complete the task and accomplish their goals.

The quality of performance is measured by standards generated by both the individual and others in the social and cultural environments in which the performance occurs. Quality is a continuum of expectations set within particular activities and contexts (Fig. 1).

UNIFORM TERMINOLOGY FOR OCCUPATIONAL THERAPY–THIRD EDITION

Occupational therapy is the use of purposeful activity or interventions to promote health and achieve functional outcomes. Achieving functional outcomes means to develop, improve, or restore the highest possible level of independence of any individual who is limited by a

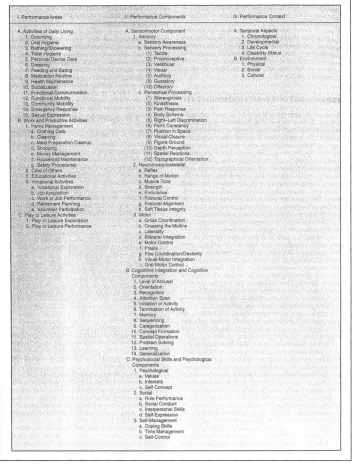

FIGURE H-1. Uniform Terminology for Occupational Therapy—Third Edition outline.

physical injury or illness, a dysfunctional condition, a cognitive impairment, a psychosocial dysfunction, a mental illness, a developmental or learning disability, or an adverse environmental condition. Assessment means the use of skilled observation or evaluation by the administration and interpretation of standardized or nonstandardized tests and measurements to identify areas for occupational therapy services. Occupational therapy services include, but are not limited to

1. the assessment, treatment, and education of or consultation with the individual, family, or other persons; or
2. interventions directed toward developing, improving, or restoring daily living skills, work readiness or work performance, play skills or leisure capacities, or enhancing educational performance skills; or
3. providing for the development, improvement, or restoration of sensorimotor, oral-motor, perceptual or neuromuscular functioning; or emotional, motivational, cognitive, or psychosocial components of performance.

These services may require assessment of the need for and use of interventions such as the design, development, adaptation, application, or training in the use of assistive technology devices; the design, fabrication, or application of rehabilitative technology such as selected orthotic devices; training in the use of assistive technology, orthotic or prosthetic devices; the application of physical agent modalities as an adjunct to or in preparation for purposeful activity; the use of ergonomic principles; the adaptation of environments and processes to enhance functional performance; or the promotion of health and wellness (AOTA, 1993, p. 1117).

I. Performance Areas

Throughout this document, activities have been described as if individuals performed the tasks themselves. Occupational therapy also recognizes that individuals arrange for tasks to be done through others. The profession views independence as the ability to self-determine activity performance, regardless of who actually performs the activity.
A. Activities of Daily Living—Self-maintenance tasks.
   1. Grooming—Obtaining and using supplies; removing body hair (use of razors, tweezers, lotions, etc.); applying and removing cosmetics; washing, drying, combing, styling, and brushing hair; caring for nails (hands and feet), caring for skin, ears, and eyes; and applying deodorant.
   2. Oral Hygiene—Obtaining and using supplies; cleaning mouth;

brushing and flossing teeth; or removing, cleaning, and reinserting dental orthotics and prosthetics.

3. Bathing/Showering—Obtaining and using supplies; soaping, rinsing, and drying body parts; maintaining bathing position; and transferring to and from bathing positions.

4. Toilet Hygiene—Obtaining and using supplies; clothing management; maintaining toileting position; transferring to and from toileting position; cleaning body; and caring for menstrual and continence needs (including catheters, colostomies, and suppository management).

5. Personal Device Care—Cleaning and maintaining personal care items, such as hearing aids, contact lenses, glasses, orthotics, prosthetics, adaptive equipment, and contraceptive and sexual devices.

6. Dressing—Selecting clothing and accessories appropriate to time of day, weather, and occasion; obtaining clothing from storage area; dressing and undressing in a sequential fashion; fastening and adjusting clothing and shoes; and applying and removing personal devices, prostheses, or orthoses.

7. Feeding and Eating—Setting up food; selecting and using appropriate utensils and tableware; bringing food or drink to mouth; cleaning face, hands, and clothing; sucking, masticating, coughing, and swallowing; and management of alternative methods of nourishment.

8. Medication Routine—Obtaining medication, opening and closing containers, following prescribed schedules, taking correct quantities, reporting problems and adverse effects, and administering correct quantities by using prescribed methods.

9. Health Maintenance—Developing and maintaining routines for illness prevention and wellness promotion, such as physical fitness, nutrition, and decreasing health risk behaviors.

10. Socialization—Accessing opportunities and interacting with other people in appropriate contextual and cultural ways to meet emotional and physical needs.

11. Functional Communication—Using equipment or systems to send and receive information, such as writing equipment, telephones, typewriters, computers, communication boards, call lights, emergency systems, Braille writers, telecommunication devices for the deaf, and augmentative communication systems.

12. Functional Mobility—Moving from one position or place to another, such as in-bed mobility, wheelchair mobility, transfers (wheelchair, bed, car, tub, toilet, tub/shower, chair, floor). Performing functional ambulation and transporting objects.

APPENDIX H

13. Community Mobility—Moving self in the community and using public or private transportation, such as driving, or accessing buses, taxi cabs, or other public transportation systems.
14. Emergency Response—Recognizing sudden, unexpected hazardous situations, and initiating action to reduce the threat to health and safety.
15. Sexual Expression—Engaging in desired sexual and intimate activities.

B. Work and Productive Activities—Purposeful activities for self-development, social contribution, and livelihood.

1. Home Management—Obtaining and maintaining personal and household possessions and environment.
   a. Clothing Care—Obtaining and using supplies; sorting; laundering (hand, machine, and dry clean); folding; ironing; storing; and mending.
   b. Cleaning—Obtaining and using supplies; picking up; putting away; vacuuming; sweeping and mopping floors; dusting; polishing; scrubbing; washing windows; cleaning mirrors; making beds; and removing trash and recyclables.
   c. Meal Preparation and Cleanup—Planning nutritious meals; preparing and serving food; opening and closing containers, cabinets, and drawers; using kitchen utensils and appliances; cleaning up and storing food safely.
   d. Shopping—Preparing shopping lists (grocery and other); selecting and purchasing items; selecting method of payment; and completing money transactions.
   e. Money Management—Budgeting, paying bills, and using bank systems.
   f. Household Maintenance—Maintaining home, yard, garden, appliances, vehicles, and household items.
   g. Safety Procedures—Knowing and performing preventive and emergency procedures to maintain a safe environment and to prevent injuries.
2. Care of Others—Providing for children, spouse, parents, pets, or others, such as giving physical care, nurturing, communicating, and using age-appropriate activities.
3. Educational Activities—Participating in a learning environment through school, community, or work-sponsored activities, such as exploring educational interests, attending to instruction, managing assignments, and contributing to group experiences.
4. Vocational Activities—Participating in work-related activities.
   a. Vocational Exploration—Determining aptitudes; develop-

ing interests and skills, and selecting appropriate vocational pursuits.

   b. Job Acquisition—Identifying and selecting work opportunities, and completing application and interview processes.

   c. Work or Job Performance—Performing job tasks in a timely and effective manner; incorporating necessary work behaviors.

   d. Retirement Planning—Determining aptitudes; developing interests and skills; and selecting appropriate avocational pursuits.

   e. Volunteer Participation—Performing unpaid activities for the benefit of selected individuals, groups, or causes.

C. Play or Leisure Activities—Intrinsically motivating activities for amusement, relaxation, spontaneous enjoyment, or self-expression.

   1. Play or Leisure Exploration—Identifying interests, skills, opportunities, and appropriate play or leisure activities.

   2. Play or Leisure Performance—Planning and participating in play or leisure activities. Maintaining a balance of play or leisure activities with work and productive activities, and activities of daily living. Obtaining, utilizing, and maintaining equipment and supplies.

II. Performance Components

A. Sensorimotor Component—The ability to receive input, process information, and produce output.

   1. Sensory

      a. Sensory Awareness—Receiving and differentiating sensory stimuli.

      b. Sensory Processing—Interpreting sensory stimuli:

         (1) Tactile—Interpreting light touch, pressure, temperature, pain, and vibration through skin contact/receptors.

         (2) Proprioceptive—Interpreting stimuli originating in muscles, joints, and other internal tissues that give information about the position of one body part in relation to another.

         (3) Vestibular—Interpreting stimuli from the inner ear receptors regarding head position and movement.

         (4) Visual—Interpreting stimuli through the eyes, including peripheral vision and acuity, and awareness of color and pattern.

APPENDIX H

    (5) Auditory—Interpreting and localizing sounds, and discriminating background sounds.

    (6) Gustatory—Interpreting tastes.

    (7) Olfactory—Interpreting odors.

  c. Perceptual Processing—Organizing sensory input into meaningful patterns.

    (1) Stereognosis—Identifying objects through proprioception, cognition, and the sense of touch.

    (2) Kinesthesia—Identifying the excursion and direction of joint movement.

    (3) Pain Response—Interpreting noxious stimuli.

    (4) Body Scheme—Acquiring an internal awareness of the body and the relationship of body parts to each other.

    (5) Right–Left Discrimination—Differentiating one side from the other

    (6) Form Constancy—Recognizing forms and objects as the same in various environments, positions, and sizes.

    (7) Position in Space—Determining the spatial relationship of figures and objects to self or other forms and objects.

    (8) Visual-Closure—Identifying forms or objects from incomplete presentations.

    (9) Figure Ground—Differentiating between foreground and background forms and objects.

    (10) Depth Perception—Determining the relative distance between objects, figures, or landmarks and the observer, and changes in planes of surfaces.

    (11) Spatial Relations—Determining the position of objects relative to each other.

    (12) Topographical Orientation—Determining the location of objects and settings and the route to the location.

2. Neuromusculoskeletal

  a. Reflex—Eliciting an involuntary muscle response by sensory input.

  b. Range of Motion—Moving body parts through an arc.

  c. Muscle Tone—Demonstrating a degree of tension or resistance in a muscle at rest and in response to stretch.

  d. Strength—Demonstrating a degree of muscle power when movement is resisted, as with objects or gravity.

  e. Endurance—Sustaining cardiac, pulmonary, and musculoskeletal exertion over time.

  f. Postural Control—Using righting and equilibrium adjustments to maintain balance during functional movements.

g. Postural Alignment—Maintaining biomechanical integrity among body parts.

h. Soft Tissue Integrity—Maintaining anatomical and physiological condition of interstitial tissue and skin.

3. Motor

a. Gross Coordination—Using large muscle groups for controlled, goal-directed movements.

b. Crossing the Midline—Moving limbs and eyes across the midsagittal plane of the body.

c. Laterality—Using a preferred unilateral body part for activities requiring a high level of skill.

d. Bilateral Integration—Coordinating both body sides during activity.

e. Motor Control—Using the body in functional and versatile movement patterns.

f. Praxis—Conceiving and planning a new motor act in response to an environmental demand.

g. Fine Coordination/Dexterity—Using small muscle groups for controlled movements, particularly in object manipulation.

h. Visual-Motor Integration—Coordinating the interaction of information from the eyes with body movement during activity.

i. Oral-Motor Control—Coordinating oropharyngeal musculature for controlled movements.

B. Cognitive Integration and Cognitive Components—The ability to use higher brain functions.

1. Level of Arousal—Demonstrating alertness and responsiveness to environmental stimuli.

2. Orientation—Identifying person, place, time, and situation.

3. Recognition—Identifying familiar faces, objects, and other previously presented materials.

4. Attention Span—Focusing on a task over time.

5. Initiation of Activity—Starting a physical or mental activity.

6. Termination of Activity—Stopping an activity at an appropriate time.

7. Memory—Recalling information after brief or long periods of time.

8. Sequencing—Placing information, concepts, and actions in order.

9. Categorization—Identifying similarities of and differences among pieces of environmental information.

10. Concept Formation—Organizing a variety of information to form thoughts and ideas.

APPENDIX H

11. Spatial Operations—Mentally manipulating the position of objects in various relationships.

12. Problem Solving—Recognizing a problem, defining a problem, identifying alternative plans, selecting a plan, organizing steps in a plan, implementing a plan, and evaluating the outcome.

13. Learning—Acquiring new concepts and behaviors.

14. Generalization—Applying previously learned concepts and behaviors to a variety of new situations.

C. Psychosocial Skills and Psychological Components—The ability to interact in society and to process emotions.

1. Psychological

    a. Values—Identifying ideas or beliefs that are important to self and others.

    b. Interests—Identifying mental or physical activities that create pleasure and maintain attention.

    c. Self-Concept—Developing the value of the physical, emotional, and sexual self.

2. Social

    a. Role Performance—Identifying, maintaining, and balancing functions one assumes or acquires in society (e.g., worker, student, parent, friend, religious participant).

    b. Social Conduct—Interacting by using manners, personal space, eye contact, gestures, active listening, and self-expression appropriate to one's environment.

    c. Interpersonal Skills—Using verbal and nonverbal communication to interact in a variety of settings.

    d. Self-Expression—Using a variety of styles and skills to express thoughts, feelings, and needs.

3. Self-Management

    a. Coping Skills—Identifying and managing stress and related factors.

    b. Time Management—Planning and participating in a balance of self-care, work, leisure, and rest activities to promote satisfaction and health.

    c. Self-Control—Modifying one's own behavior in response to environmental needs, demands, constraints, personal aspirations, and feedback from others.

III. Performance Contexts

Assessment of function in performance areas is greatly influenced by the contexts in which the individual must perform. Occupational therapy practitioners consider performance contexts when determining feasibility and appropriateness of interventions. Occupational therapy practitioners may choose interventions based on an understanding of contexts, or may choose interventions directly aimed at altering the contexts to improve performance.

A. Temporal Aspects
1. Chronological—Individual's age.
2. Developmental—Stage or phase of maturation.
3. Life cycle—Place in important life phases, such as career cycle, parenting cycle, or educational process.
4. Disability status—Place in continuum of disability, such as acuteness of injury, chronicity of disability, or terminal nature of illness.

B. Environment
1. Physical—Nonhuman aspects of contexts. Includes the accessibility to and performance within environments having natural terrain, plants, animals, building, furniture, objects, tools, or devices.
2. Social—Availability and expectations of significant individuals, such as spouse, friends, and caregivers. Also includes larger social groups which are influential in establishing norms, role expectations, and social routines.
3. Cultural—Customs, beliefs, activity patterns, behavior standards, and expectations accepted by the society of which the individual is a member. Includes political aspects, such as laws that affect access to resources and affirm personal rights. Also includes opportunities for education, employment, and economic support.

REFERENCES

American Occupational Therapy Association. (1979). Occupational therapy product output reporting system and uniform terminology for reporting occupational therapy services. Rockville, MD: Author.

American Occupational Therapy Association. (1989). Uniform terminology for occupational therapy—Second edition. American Journal of Occupational Therapy, 43, 808–815.

American Occupational Therapy Association. (1993). Association policies—Definition of occupational therapy practice for state regulation (Policy 5.3.1). American Journal of Occupational Therapy, 47, 1117–1121.

Prepared by The Terminology Task Force: Winifred Dunn, PhD, OTR, FAOTA, Chairperson; Mary Foto, OTR, FAOTA; Jim Hinojosa, PhD, OTR, FAOTA; Barbara Schell, PhD, OTR/L, FAOTA; Linda Kohlman Thomson,

APPENDIX H

MOT, OTR, FAOTA; Sarah D. Hertfelder, MEd, MOT, OTR/L—Staff Liaison, for The Commission on Practice (Jim Hinojosa, PhD, OTR, FAOTA, Chairperson).

Adopted by the Representative Assembly July 1994.

This document replaces the following documents, all of which were rescinded by the 1994 Representative Assembly: Occupational Therapy Product Output Reporting System (1979), Uniform Terminology for Reporting Occupational Therapy Services—First Edition (1979), "Uniform Occupational Therapy Evaluation Checklist" (1981, American Journal of Occupational Therapy, 35, 817–818), and "Uniform Terminology for Occupational Therapy—Second Edition" (1989, American Journal of Occupational Therapy, 43, 808–815).

I

INTERNATIONAL CLASSIFICATION OF IMPAIRMENTS, ACTIVITIES, AND PARTICIPATION

The International Classification of Impairments, Activities, and Participation (ICIDH-2) is a revision of the International Classification of Impairments, Disability, and Handicap (ICIDH). ICIDH-2 "classifies human functioning at the level of the body, the whole person, and the person within the complete social and physical environmental context" (World Health Organization [WHO], 1998, p. 2). This new classification has moved away from terminology like "disability" and "handicap" to a terminology that more clearly identifies a person's realm of difficulty due to a disorder or disease. "Disabilities" has been replaced with "activities" and "handicap" has been replaced with "participation." ICIDH-2 also includes a list of contextual or environmental factors—both physical and social—that can influence one's abilities to engage in both activities and participation. This classification system is still being trial tested and is not yet final. Definitions for the main concepts of ICIDH-2 are listed below, from the hypertext version of Beta-2 version of ICIDH-2 (WHO, 1999). For updates on this terminology, see www.who.int/icidh

BODY FUNCTIONS

Body functions are the physiological or psychological functions of body systems. Impairments are problems in body function or structure as a significant deviation or loss.

BODY STRUCTURE

Body structures are anatomical parts of the body such as organs, limbs, and their components. Impairments are problems in body function or structure as a significant deviation or loss.

ACTIVITIES

Activity is the performance of a task or action by an individual. Activity limitations are difficulties in performance of activities.

PARTICIPATION

Participation is an individual's involvement in life situations in relation to Health Conditions, Body Functions or Structures, Activities, and Contextual Factors. Participation Restrictions are problems an individual may have in the manner or extent of involvement in life situations.

ENVIRONMENTAL FACTORS

Environmental factors make up the physical, social, and attitudinal environment in which people live and conduct their lives.

REFERENCES

Allen, C. K. (1985). *Occupational therapy for psychiatric diseases: Measurement and management of cognitive disabilities.* Boston: Little, Brown and Co.

Allen, C. K. (1990). *Allen cognitive level test manual.* Colchester, CT: S & S Worldwide.

Allen, C. K. (1992). Cognitive disabilities. In N. Katz (Ed.), *Cognitive rehabilitation. Models of intervention in occupational therapy* (pp. 1–21). Stoneham, MA: Butterworth-Heinemann.

Allen, C. K. (1996). *Allen Cognitive Level Screen. Test manual.* Colchester, CT: S & S Worldwide.

Allen, C. K. (1998). Cognitive disability frame of reference. In M. E. Neistadt & E. B. Crepeau (Eds.), *Willard & Spackman's occupational therapy* (pp. 555–557). Philadelphia: Lippincott.

Allen, C. K., Earhart, C. A., & Blue, T. (1992). *Occupational therapy treatment goals for the physically and cognitively challenged.* Rockville, MD: American Occupational Therapy Association.

Allen, C. K., Kehrberg, K., & Burns, T. (1992). Evaluation instruments. In C. K. Allen, C. A. Earhart, & T. Blue (Eds.), *Occupational therapy treatment goals for the physically and cognitively challenged* (pp. 31–68). Rockville, MD: American Occupational Therapy Association.

American College of Sports Medicine (1991). *Guidelines for exercise testing and prescription* (4th ed.). Philadelphia: Lea & Febiger.

American Occupational Therapy Association (1994). Uniform terminology for occupational therapy—3rd edition. *American Journal of Occupational Therapy, 48,* 1047–1054.

Árnadóttir, G. (1990). *The brain and behavior: Assessing cortical dysfunction through tasks of daily living.* St. Louis: The C.V. Mosby Co.

Ashworth, B. (1964). Preliminary trial of carisoprodol in multiple sclerosis. *Practitioner, 192,* 540–542.

Asmussen, E. (1979). Muscle fatigue. *Medical Science and Sports, 11,* 313–321.

Atchison, B. (1995). Cardiopulmonary diseases. In C. A. Trombly (Ed.), *Occupational therapy for physical dysfunction* (4th ed.) (pp. 875–892). Philadelphia: Williams & Wilkins.

Barrows, H. (1980). *Guide to neurological assessment.* Philadelphia: Lippincott.

Basmajian, J. V., & DeLuca, C. J. (1985). *Muscles alive: Their functions revealed by electromyography* (5th ed.). Baltimore: Williams & Wilkins.

Baron, K., Kielhofner, G., Goldhammer, V., & Wolenski, J. (1998). *A user's manual for the Occupational Self-Assessment (OSA) (Version 1.0).* Chicago: University of Illinois at Chicago.

Barris, R., Dickie, V., & Baron, K. B. (1988). A comparison of psychiatric patients and normal subjects based on the model of human occupation. *Occupational Therapy Journal of Research, 8,* 3–37.

Barris, R., Kielhofner, G., Burch, R. M., Gelinas, I., Klement, M., & Schultz, B. (1986). Occupational function and dysfunction in three groups of adolescents. *Occupational Therapy Journal of Research, 6,* 301–317.

Barris, R., Oakley, F., & Kielhofner, G. (1988). The role checklist. In B. Hemphill (Ed.), *Mental health assessment in occupational therapy. An integrative approach to the evaluation process* (pp. 73–91). Thorofare, NJ: Slack Inc.

Bentzel, K. (1995). Evaluation of sensation. In C. A. Trombly (Ed.), *Occupational therapy for physical dysfunction* (4th ed.) (pp. 187–199). Philadelphia: Williams & Wilkins.

Berg, K., Wood-Dauphinee, S., & Williams, J. (1989). Measuring balance in the elderly. Preliminary development of an instrument. *Physiotherapy Canada, 41,* 304–311.

Biernacki, S. D. (1993). Reliability of the worker role interview. *American Journal of Occupational Therapy, 47,* 797–803.

Black, M. M. (1976). Adolescent role assessment. *American Journal of Occupational Therapy, 30,* 73–79.

Black, M. M. (1982). Adolescent role assessment. In B. Hemphill (Ed.), *The evaluative process in psychiatric occupational therapy* (pp. 49–53). Thorofare, NJ: Slack Inc.

Bobath, B. (1978). *Adult hemiplegia: Evaluation and treatment* (2nd ed.). London: William Heinemann Medical Books LTD.

Bohannon, R., & Smith M. (1987). Interrater reliability of a modified Ashworth scale of muscle spasticity. *Physical Therapy, 87,* 206–207.

Brannon, F. J., Foley, M. W., Starr, J. A., & Black, M. G. (1993). *Cardiopulmonary rehabilitation: Basic theory and application* (2nd ed.). Philadelphia: F.A. Davis.

Brennan, J. (1959, March). Clinical method of assessing tonus and voluntary movement in hemiplegia. *British Medical Journal, 21,* 767–768.

Brollier, C., Watts, J. H., Bauer, D., & Schmidt, W. (1988). A concurrent validity study of two occupational therapy evaluation instruments. The AOF and OCAIRS. *Occupational Therapy in Mental Health, 8*(4), 49–60.

Clark, F. (1993). Eleanor Clarke Slagle Lectureship—1993; Occupation embedded in a real life: Interweaving occupational science and occupational therapy. *American Journal of Occupational Therapy, 47,* 1067–1078.

Crutchfield, C., Shumway-Cook, A., & Horak, F. (1989). Balance and coordination training. In R. Skully & M. Barnes (Eds.), *Physical therapy* (825–843). Philadelphia: Lippincott.

Daniels, L., & Worthingham, C. (1986). *Muscle testing—techniques of manual examination* (5th ed.). Philadelphia: Saunders.

Dehn, M. M. (1980, March). Rehabilitation of the cardiac patient: The effects of exercise. *American Journal of Nursing, 80,* 435–440.

Dehn, M. M., & Mullins, C. B. (1977, April). Physiologic effects and importance of exercise in patients with coronary artery disease. *Cardiovascular Medicine, 2,* 365–371 & 377–387.

DiFablo, R. P., & Badke, M. B. (1990). Relationship of sensory organization to balance function in patients with hemiplegia. *Physical Therapy, 70,* 342–548.

Doble, S. E., Fisk, J. D., Fisher, A. G., Ritvo, P. G., & Murray, T. J. (1994). Functional competence of community-dwelling persons with multiple sclerosis using the Assessment of Motor and Process Skills. *Archives of Physical Medicine and Rehabilitation, 75,* 843–851.

Duncan, P., Weiner, D., Chandler, J., & Studenski, S. (1990). Functional reach: A new clinical measure of balance. *Journal of Gerontology: Medical Sciences, 45*(6), 192–197.

Dunn, W. (1991). Assessing sensory performance enablers. In C. Christiansen & C. Baum (Eds.), *Occupational Therapy. Overcoming human performance deficits* (pp. 471–505). Thorofare, NJ: Slack Inc.

Ebb, E. W., Coster, W., & Duncombe, L. (1989). Comparison of normal and psychosocially dysfunctional male adolescents. *Occupational Therapy in Mental Health, 9*(2), 53–74.

Elazar, B., Itzkovich, M., & Katz, N. (1996). *Lowenstein Occupational Therapy Cognitive Assessment for Geriatric Population (LOTCA-G) manual.* Printed in the United States.

Farber, S. D. (1991a). Assessing neuromotor performance enablers. In C. Christiansen & C. Baum (Eds.), *Occupational therapy. Overcoming human performance deficits* (pp. 507–521). Thorofare, NJ: Slack Inc.

Farber S. D. (1991b). Neuromotor dimensions of performance. In C. Christiansen & C. Baum (Eds.), *Occupational therapy. Overcoming human performance deficits* (pp. 259–282). Thorofare, NJ: Slack Inc.

Fess, E. E. (1993). Hand rehabilitation. In H. L. Hopkins & H. D. Smith (Eds.), *Willard & Spackman's occupational therapy* (8th ed.) (pp. 674–690). Philadelphia: Lippincott.

Fillenbaum, G. G. (1988). *Multidimensional functional assessment of older adults: The Duke older Americans resources and services procedures.* Hillsdale, NJ: Lawrence Erlbaum Associates.

Fisher, A. G. (1994). Assessment of motor and process skills manual (research edition 7.0). [Unpublished test manual]. Fort Collins: Colorado State University.

Fisher, A. G., Liu, Y., Velozo, C. A., & Pan, A. W. (1992). Cross-cultural assessment of process skills. *American Journal of Occupational Therapy, 46,* 876–885.

Folstein, M. F., Folstein, S. F., & McHugh, P. R. (1975). Mini-Mental State. A practical method for grading the cognitive state of patients for the clinician. *Journal of Psychiatric Research, 12,* 189–198.

Fugl-Meyer, A., Jaasko, L., Leyman, I., Olson, S., & Steglind, S. (1975). The post-stroke hemiplegic patient: a method for evaluation of physical performance. *Scandinavian Journal of Rehabilitation Medicine, 7,* 13–31.

Gilfoyle, E. M., Grady, A. P., & Moore, J. C. (1981). *Children adapt*. Thorofare, NJ: Slack Inc.

Golden (1978). *Stroop Color and Word Test. A manual for clinical and experimental uses*. Wood Dale, IL: Stoelting Company.

Good-Ellis, M. A., Fine S. B., Hass, G. L., Spencer, J. H., & Glick, I. D. (1986). Quantitative role and performance assessment: Implications and application to treatment of major affective disorders. In *Depression: Assessment and treatment update*. Proceedings from the AOTA Preconference Institute to the American Psychiatric Association's Institute on Hospital and Community Psychiatry. Rockville, MD: AOTA.

Good-Ellis, M. A., Fine, S. B., Spencer, J. H., & DiVittis, A. (1987). Developing a role activity performance scale. *American Journal of Occupational Therapy, 41*, 232–241.

Gregory, M. (1983). Occupational behavior and life satisfaction among retirees. *American Journal of Occupational Therapy, 37*, 548–552.

Gurland, B., Kuriansky, J., Sharpe, L., Simon, R., Stiller, P., & Birkett, P. (1977–78). The Comprehensive Assessment and Referral Evaluation (CARE). *International Journal of Aging and Human Development, 8*, 9–42.

Hamilton, B. B., Granger, C. V., Sherwin, F. S., Zielezny, M., & Tashman, J. S. (1987). A uniform national data system for medical rehabilitation. In M. J. Fuhrer (Ed.), *Rehabilitation outcomes: Analysis and measurement* (pp. 137–147). Baltimore: Paul H. Brooks Publishing Co.

Handelsman, D. (1994). *The construct validity of the worker role interview for the chronic mentally ill*. Unpublished master's thesis, University of Illinois at Chicago.

Hartman-Maeir, A., & Katz, N. (1995). Validity of the Behavioral Inattention Test (BIT): Relationships with functional tasks. *American Journal of Occupational Therapy, 49*, 507–516.

Heaton, R. K., Chelune, G. J., Talley, J. L., Kay, G. G., & Curtiss, G. (1993). *Wisconsin Card Sorting Test manual*. Odessa, FL: Psychological Assessment Resources, Incorporated.

Heimann, N. E., Allen, C. K., & Yerxa, E. J. (1989). The Routine Task Inventory: A tool for describing the functional behavior of the cognitively disabled. *Occupational Therapy Practice, 1*, 67–74.

Heinemann, A. W., Linacre, J. M., Wright, B. D., Hamilton, B. B., & Granger, C. (1994). Prediction of rehabilitation outcomes with disability measures. *Archives of Physical Medicine and Rehabilitation, 75*, 133–143.

Henry, A. D. (1994). *Predicting psychosocial functioning and symptomatic recovery of adolescents and young adults with a first psychotic episode: A six-month follow-up study*. Unpublished doctoral dissertation, Boston University.

Henry, A. (1996, April). *Development of a measure of adolescent leisure interests*. Poster presentation of the American Occupational Therapy Association Annual Conference, Chicago, IL.

Henry, A. D. (1998). The interview process in occupational therapy. In M. E. Neistadt & E. B. Crepeau (Eds.), *Willard & Spackman's occupational therapy* (9th ed.) (pp. 155–168). Philadelphia: Lippincott.

Henry, A. D., & Mallinson, T. (1999). The Occupational Performance History Interview. In B. J. Hemphill (Ed.), *Assessments in occupational therapy mental health. An integrative approach* (pp. 59–70). Thorofare, NJ: Slack Inc.

Henry, A. D., Moore, K., Quinlivan, M., & Triggs, M. (1998). The relationship of the Allen Cognitive Level Test to demographics, diagnosis, and disposition among psychiatric inpatients. *American Journal of Occupational Therapy, 52*, 638–643.

Hooper, H. E. (1985). *The Hooper Visual Organization Test.* Los Angeles: Western Psychological Services.

Ilika, J., & Hoffman, N. G. (1981a). *Reliability study on the Kohlman Evaluation of Living Skills.* Unpublished manuscript.

Ilika, J., & Hoffman, N. G. (1981b). *Concurrent validity study on the Kohlman Evaluation of Living Skills and the Global Assessment Scale.* Unpublished manuscript.

Itzkovich, M., Elazar, B., Averbuch, S., & Katz, N. (1990). *Lowenstein Occupational Therapy Cognitive Assessment (LOTCA) manual.* Printed in the United States.

Jaworski, D. M., Kult, T., & Boynton, P. R. (1994). The Functional Independence Measure: A pilot study comparison of observed and reported ratings. *Rehabilitation Nursing Research, Winter,* 141–147.

Jebsen, R. H., Taylor, N., Trieschmann, R. B., Trotter, M. J., & Howard, L. A. (1969). An objective and standardized test of hand function. *Archives of Physical Medicine and Rehabilitation, 50,* 311–319.

Kaplan, K., & Kielhofner, G. (1989). *Occupational case analysis interview and rating scale.* Thorofare, NJ: Slack Inc.

Kaufman, L. (1982). *Concurrent validity study on the Kohlman Evaluation of Living Skills and the Bay Area Functional Performance Evaluation.* Unpublished master's thesis, University of Florida, Gainesville.

Kendall, F. P., McCreary, E. K., & Provance, P. G. (1993). *Muscles testing and function* (4th ed). Baltimore: Williams & Wilkins.

Kielhofner, G. (Ed.) (1985). *A model of human occupation. Theory and application.* Baltimore: Williams & Wilkins.

Kielhofner, G. (Ed.) (1995). *A model of human occupation. Theory and application.* (2nd ed.). Baltimore: Williams & Wilkins.

Kielhofner, G., Mallinson, T., Crawford, C., Nowak, M., Rigby, M., Henry, A., & Walens, D. (1998). *A user's manual for the Occupational Performance History Interview* (2nd version). Chicago: Model of Human Occupational Clearing House, University of Illinois at Chicago.

Kielhofner, G., & Neville, A. (1983). *The modified interest checklist.* Unpublished manuscript, University of Illinois at Chicago.

Klein, R. M., & Bell, B. (1979). *The Klein-Bell ADL Scale Manual. Seattle,* WA: Educational Resources, University of Washington.

Klein, R. M., & Bell, B. (1982). Self-care skills: Behavioral measurement with Klein-Bell ADL scale. *Archives of Physical Medicine and Rehabilitation, 63,* 335–338.

Kohlmeyer, K. (1998). Evaluation of sensory and neuromuscular performance components. In M. E. Neistadt & E. B. Crepeau (Eds.), *Willard & Spackman's occupational therapy* (9th ed.) (pp. 223–260). Philadelphia: Lippincott.

Lamb, R. (1985). Manual muscle testing. In Rothstein (Ed.), *Measurement in physical therapy* (pp. 47–55). New York: Churchill-Livingstone.

LaStays, P., & Wheeler, D. (1994). Reliability of passive wrist flexion and extension goniometric measurements: a multicenter study. *Physical Therapy, 74,* 162–174.

Law, M., Baptiste, S., Carswell, A., McColl, M. A., Polatajko, H., & Pollock, N. (1998). *Canadian occupational performance measure* (3rd ed.). Ottawa, Canada: CAOT Publications ACE.

Lawton, M. P. & Brody, E. M. (1969). Assessment of older people: self maintaining and instrumental activities of daily living. *Gerontologist, 9,* 179–186.

Leonardelli, C. A. (1988a). *The Milwaukee Evaluation of Daily Living Skills.* Thorofare, NJ: Slack Inc.

Leonardelli, C. A. (1988b). The Milwaukee Evaluation of Daily Living Skills (MEDLS). In B. J. Hemphill (Ed.), *Mental health assessment in occupational therapy* (pp. 151–162). Thorofare, NJ: Slack Inc.

Linacre, J. M. (1989). *Many-facet Rasch measurement.* Chicago: MESA Press.

Linacre, J. M., Heinemann, A. W., Wright, B. D., Granger, C. V., & Hamilton, B. B. (1994). The structure and stability of the Functional Independence Measure. *Archives of Physical Medicine and Rehabilitation, 75,* 127–132.

Lunsford, B. R. (1978). Clinical indicators of endurance. *Physical Therapy, 58,* 704–709.

Markos, P. (1977). *Comparison of hold-relax and contract-relax and contralateral effects.* Unpublished master's thesis, Boston University.

Mathiowetz, V., & Haugen, J. B. (1995). Evaluation of motor behavior: Traditional and contemporary views. In C. A. Trombly (Ed.), *Occupational therapy for physical dysfunction* (4th ed.) (pp. 157–185). Philadelphia: Williams & Wilkins.

Mathiowetz, V., Volland, G., Kashman, N., & Weber, K. (1985). Adult norms for the box and block test of manual dexterity. *American Journal of Occupational Therapy, 39,* 386–391.

Mathiowetz, V., Weber, K., Kashman, N., & Volland, G. (1985). Adult norms for the nine-hole peg test of finger dexterity. *Occupational Therapy Journal of Research, 5,* 24–38.

Matsutsuyu, J. (1969). The interest checklist. *American Journal of Occupational Therapy, 23,* 323–328.

Mattingly, C., & Fleming, M. H. (1994). *Clinical reasoning: Forms of inquiry in a therapeutic practice.* Philadelphia: F.A. Davis.

McGourty, L. K. (1979). *Kohlman Evaluation of Living Skills.* Seattle, WA: KELS Research.

McGourty, L. K. (1988). Kohlman Evaluation of Living Skills. In B. Hemphill (Ed.), *Mental health assessment in occupational therapy* (pp. 133–146). Thorofare, NJ: Slack Inc.

Miller, R., Groher, M., Yorkston, K., & Rees, T (1988). Speech, language, swallowing and auditory rehabilitation. In J. DeLisa (Ed.), *Rehabilitation medicine principles and practice* (pp. 116–139). Philadelphia: Lippincott.

Minor, M. (1991). Assessing the physiological enablers of performance. In C. Christiansen & C. Baum (Eds.), *Occupational therapy. Overcoming human performance deficits* (pp. 455–468). Thorofare, NJ: Slack Inc.

Neistadt, M. E. (1992). The Rabideau Kitchen Evaluation—Revised: An assessment of meal preparation skill. *Occupational Therapy Journal of Research, 12,* 242–255.

Neistadt, M. E. (1996). Teaching strategies for the development of clinical reasoning. *American Journal of Occupational Therapy, 50,* 676–684.

Neistadt, M. E. (1998). Teaching clinical reasoning as a thinking frame. *American Journal of Occupational Therapy, 52,* 221–229.

Neistadt, M. E., & Crepeau, E. B. (1998). Introduction to occupational therapy. In M. E. Neistadt & E. B. Crepeau (Eds.), *Willard & Spackman's occupational therapy* (9th ed.) (pp. 5–12). Philadelphia: Lippincott.

Nelson, K. L. (1996). Dysphagia: Evaluation and treatment. In L. W. Pedretti (Ed.), *Occupational therapy. Practice skills for physical dysfunction* (4th ed.) (pp. 165–191). St. Louis: C.V. Mosby Co.

Nygård, L., Bernspång, B., Fisher, A. G., & Winblad, B. (1994). Comparing motor and process ability of persons with suspected dementia in home and clinic settings. *American Journal of Occupational Therapy, 48,* 689–696.

Oakley, F., Kielhofner, G., Barris, R., & Reichler, R. (1986). The role checklist: Development and empirical assessment of reliability. *Occupational Therapy Journal of Research, 6,* 157–170.

Okkema, K. (1993a). *Cognition and perception in the stroke patient.* Gaithersburg, MD: Aspen Publishers, Inc.

Pedretti, L. W. (1996a). Evaluation of joint range of motion. In L. W. Pedretti (Ed.), *Occupational therapy. Practice skills for physical dysfunction* (4th ed.) (pp. 79–107). St. Louis: C.V. Mosby Co.

Pedretti, L. W. (1996b). Evaluation of muscle strength. In L. W. Pedretti (Ed.), *Occupational therapy. Practice skills for physical dysfunction* (4th ed.) (pp. 109–149). St. Louis: C.V. Mosby Co.

Pedretti, L. W. (1996c). Evaluation of sensation and treatment of sensory dysfunction. In L. W. Pedretti (Ed.), *Occupational therapy. Practice skills for physical dysfunction* (4th ed.) (pp. 213–230). St. Louis: C.V. Mosby Co.

Pfeffer, R. I., Kurosaki, T. T., Harrah, C. H., Chance, J. M., & Filos, S. (1982). Measurement of functional activities in older adults in the community. *Journal of Gerontology, 37,* 323–329.

Rabideau, G. M. (1986). *Two approaches to improving the functional performance of a cognitively impaired head injured adult.* Master's thesis. (Available from Tufts University, Medford, MA 02155).

Rancho (1978). *Guide for muscle testing of the upper extremity.* Rancho Los

Amigos Hospital Occupational Therapy Department. Downey, CA: Professional Staff Association of Rancho Los Amigos Hospital, Inc.

Riddle, D. (1992). Measurement of accessory motion: Critical issues and related concepts. *Physical Therapy, 72,* 865–874.

Rogers, J. C. (1983). Clinical reasoning: The ethics, science, and art, 1983 Eleanor Clarke Slagle Lecture. *American Journal of Occupational Therapy, 37,* 601–616.

Rogers, J. C. (1985). Articulating a frame of reference in occupational therapy. In M. Kirkland & S. C. Robertson (Eds.), *Planning and implementing vocational readiness in occupational therapy* (pp. 137–145). Rockville, MD: American Occupational Therapy Association.

Rogers, J. C. (1988). The NPI Interest Checklist. In B. J. Hemphill (Ed.), *Mental health assessment in occupational therapy. An integrative approach to the evaluation process.* Thorofare, NJ: Slack Inc.

Rogers, J. C., & Holm, M. B. (1989). Performance Assessment of Self-Care Skills-Revised (PASS-R). Unpublished functional performance test. Pittsburgh, PA: University of Pittsburgh.

Rogers, J. C., & Holm, M. B. (1994). Performance Assessment of Self-Care Skills (PASS) (version 3.1). Unpublished functional performance test. Pittsburgh, PA: University of Pittsburgh.

Rogers, J. C., & Holm, M. B. (1998). Evaluation of Activities of Daily Living (ADL) and home management. In M. E. Neistadt & E. B. Crepeau (Eds.), *Willard & Spackman's occupational therapy* (9th ed.) (pp. 185–208). Philadelphia: Lippincott.

Rogers, J. C., & Masagatani, G. (1982). Clinical reasoning of occupational therapists during the initial assessment of physically disabled patients. *Occupational Therapy Journal of Research, 2,* 195–219.

Rothstein, J. M., Roy, S. H., & Wolf, S. L. (1998). *The rehabilitation specialist's handbook* (2nd ed.). Philadelphia: F.A. Davis.

Scheiman, M. (1997). *Understanding and managing vision deficits.* Thorofare, NJ: Slack.

Schell, B. B. (1998). Clinical reasoning: The basis of practice. In M. E. Neistadt & E. B. Crepeau (Eds.), *Willard & Spackman's occupational therapy* (9th ed.) (pp. 90–100). Philadelphia: Lippincott.

Schell, B. A., & Cervero, R. M. (1993). Clinical reasoning in occupational therapy: An integrative review. *American Journal of Occupational Therapy, 47,* 605–610.

Shillam, L. L., Beeman, C., & Loshin, P. M. (1983). Effect of occupational therapy intervention on bathing independence of disabled persons. *American Journal of Occupational Therapy, 37,* 744–748.

Simon, C. J., & Daub, M. M. (1993). Human development across the life span. In H. L. Hopkins & H. D. Smith (Eds.), *Willard & Spackman's occupational therapy* (8th ed.) (pp. 95–130). Philadelphia: Lippincott.

Smidt, G., & Roger M. (1982). Factors contributing to the regulation and clinical assessment of muscle strength. *Physical Therapy, 62,* 1283.

Smith, H. (1993). Assessment and evaluation: An overview. In H. L. Hopkins & H. D. Smith (Eds.), *Willard & Spackman's occupational therapy* (8th ed.) (pp. 169–191). Philadelphia: Lippincott.

Smith, N. R., Kielhofner, G., & Watts, J. H. (1986). The relationship between volition, activity pattern, and life satisfaction in the elderly. *American Journal of Occupational Therapy, 40,* 278–283.

Smyntek, L., Barris, R., & Kielhofner, G. (1985). The model of human occupation applied to psychosocially functional and dysfunctional adolescents. *Occupational Therapy in Mental Health, 5*(1), 21–40.

Spencer, J. C. (1998). Evaluation of performance contexts. In M. E. Neistadt & E. B. Crepeau (Eds.), *Willard & Spackman's occupational therapy* (9th ed.) (pp. 291–309). Philadelphia: Lippincott.

Sroufe, L. A., Cooper, R. G., & Deltart, G. B. (1992). *Child development* (2nd ed.). New York: McGraw-Hill.

Tinetti, M. E. (1986). Performance oriented assessment of mobility problems on elderly patients. *Journal of the American Geriatrics Society, 34,* 119–126.

Toglia, J. P. (1993). *Contextual Memory Test.* San Antonio, TX: Therapy Skill Builders.

Trombly, C. A. (1989). Cardiopulmonary rehabilitation. In C. A. Trombly (Ed.), *Occupational therapy for physical dysfunction* (3rd ed.) (pp. 581–603). Baltimore: Williams & Wilkins.

Trombly, C. A. (1995). Evaluation of biomechanical and physiological aspects of motor performance. In C. A. Trombly (Ed.), *Occupational therapy for physical dysfunction* (4th ed.) (pp. 73–156). Baltimore: Williams & Wilkins.

Trombly, C. A., & Quintana, L. A. (1989). Activities of daily living. In C. A. Trombly (Ed.), *Occupational therapy for physical dysfunction* (3rd ed.) (pp. 386–410). Baltimore: Williams & Wilkins.

Trombly, C. A., & Scott, A. D. (1989). Evaluation of motor control. In C. A. Trombly (Ed.) (1989). *Occupational therapy for physical dysfunction* (3rd ed.) (pp. 55–71). Baltimore: Williams & Wilkins.

Trombly, C. A., & Scott, A. D. (1989). Evaluation. In C. A. Trombly (Ed.), *Occupational therapy for physical dysfunction* (3rd ed.)(pp. 184–286). Baltimore: Williams & Wilkins.

Undzis, M. F., Zoltan, B., & Pedretti, L. W. (1996). Evaluation of motor control. In L. W. Pedretti (Ed.), *Occupational therapy. Practice skills for physical dysfunction* (4th ed.) (pp. 151–164). St. Louis: C.V. Mosby Co.

Uniform Data System for Medical Rehabilitation (UDSMR) (1997). *Guide for the uniform data set for medical rehabilitation* (including the adult FIM) (*Version 5.1*). Buffalo: State University of New York at Buffalo.

Velozo, C., Kielhofner, G., & Fisher, G. (1992). *A user's guide to the worker role interview* (Research version). University of Illinois at Chicago: Department of Occupational Therapy.

Warren, M. (1991). Strategies for sensory and neuromotor remediation. In C. Christiansen & C. Baum (Eds.), *Occupational therapy. Overcoming human performance deficits* (pp. 633–662). Thorofare, NJ: Slack Inc.

Watts, J. H., Brollier, C., Bauer, D., & Schmidt, W. (1988a). A comparison of two evaluation instruments used with psychiatric patients in occupational therapy. *Occupational Therapy in Mental Health, 8*(4), 7–27.

Watts, J. H., Brollier, C., Bauer, D., & Schmidt, W. (1988b). The assessment of occupational functioning: The second revision. *Occupational Therapy in Mental Health, 8*(4), 7–27.

Watts, J. H., Kielhofner, G., Bauer, D., Gregory, M., & Valentine, D. (1986). The assessment of occupational functioning: A screening tool for use in long-term care. *American Journal of Occupational Therapy, 40,* 231–240.

Wei, S., McQuade, K., & Smidt, G. (1993). Three-dimensional joint range of motion measurements from skeletal coordinate data. *Journal of Physical Therapy, 18,* 687–691.

Weinstein, J. (1979). *The generation of profiles of adolescent interests.* Unpublished master's thesis, University of Southern California, Los Angeles.

Western Psychological Services (1983). *Hooper Visual Organization Test (VOT) manual.* Los Angeles: Author.

Williams, J. H., Drinka, T. J. K., Greenberg, J. R., Farrel-Holtan, J., Euhardy, R., & Schram, M. (1991). Development and testing of the Assessment of Living Skills and Resources (ALSAR) in elderly community-dwelling veterans. *Gerontologist, 31,* 84–91.

Wilson, B., Cockburn, J., & Baddely, A. (1987). *The Behavioral Inattention Test.* Bury St. Edmonds: Thames Valley Test Co.

Wilson, D. S., Allen C. K., McCormack, G., & Burton, G. (1989). Cognitive disability and routine task behaviors in a community based population with senile dementia. *Occupational Therapy Practice, 1,* 58–66.

World Health Organization (WHO). (1980). *Towards a common language for functioning and disablement: ICIDH-2. The International Classification of Impairments, Activities, and Participation.* Geneva: World Health Organization.

World Health Organization (WHO). (1998). *International classification of impairments, disabilities, and handicaps: A manual of classification relating to the consequences of disease.* Geneva: World Health Organization.

World Health Organization (WHO). (1999). Hypertext version of Beta-2 version of ICIDH-2. Geneva: World Health Organization. http//:www.who.int/icidh

Worley, J., Bennett, W., Miller, G., Miller, M., Walker, B., & Harmon, C. (1991). Reliability of three clinical measures of muscle tone in the shoulders and wrists of post-stroke patients. *American Journal of Occupational Therapy, 45,* 50–58.

Yerxa, E. J., Burnett-Beaulieu, S., Stocking, S., & Azen, S. P. (1988). Development of the satisfaction with scaled performance questionnaire (SPSQ). *American Journal of Occupational Therapy, 42,* 215–222.

Zoltan (1996). *Vision, perception, and cognition. A manual for the evaluation and treatment of the neurologically impaired adult* (3rd ed.). Thorofare, NJ: Slack Inc.

Zoltan, B., Siev, E., & Freishtat, B. (1986). *Perceptual and cognitive dysfunction in the adult stroke patient.* Thorofare, NJ: Slack Inc.

Website Addresses for Organizations and Agencies Related to Evaluation

Website Address	Organization	Type of Information Available
www.aota.org	American Occupational Therapy Association	For updates on legislative issues related to occupational therapy evaluation and pubications related to evaluation
www.easy-living.com	Smith Nephew	To order assessments and evaluation equipment
www.hbtpc.com	Therapy Skill Builders	To order assessments
www.mosby.com	The C.V. Mosby Co.	For evaluation publications
www.ncmedical.com	North Coast Medical	To order assessments and evaluation equipment
www.nlm.nih.gov/ medlineplus/ medlineplus	Medlineplus, a service of the National Library of Medicine, US	For information about various health problems and access to government agencies, with links to related non-government organizations
www.parinc.com	Psychological Assessment Resources (PAR)	To order assessments
www.sammons-preston.com	Sammons Preston	To order assessments and evaluation equipment
www.slackinc.com	Slack Inc.	For evaluation publications
www.sns.wwide.com	S & S Worldwide	To order Allen Cognitive Level assessments
www.udsmr.org	Uniform Data System for Medical Rehabilitation	For information about the Functional Independence Measure (FIM)
www.uic.edu/hsc/ acad/cahp/OT/ MOHOC/	Model of Human Occupation Clearinghouse	For evaluation publications
www.who.org	World Health Organization (WHO)	For information about various health problems worldwide and WHO publications
www.who.int/icidh	World Health Organization	Information on World Health Organization's ICIDH-2
www.wpspublish.com	Western Psychological Services	To order assessments

INDEX

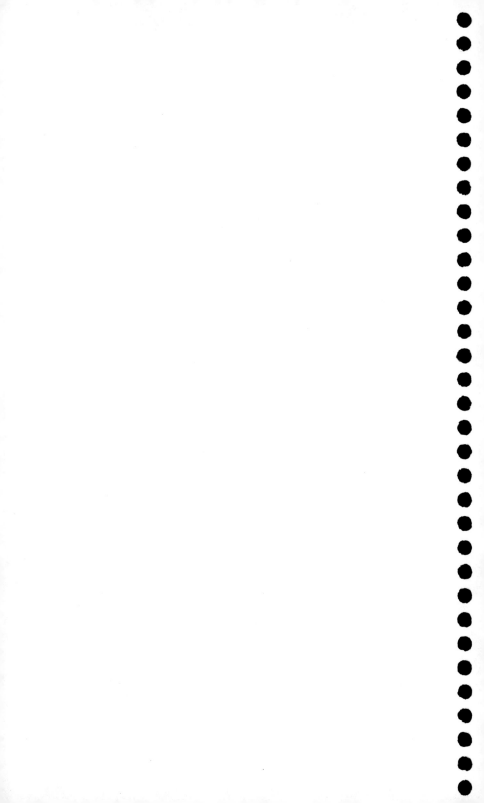